FORGET DIETS!

Your Weight Doesn't Matter But Your Food Habits Do

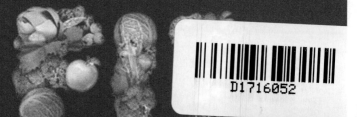

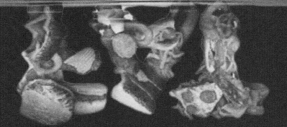

MATTHIAS STUBER

FORGET DIETS!

Your Weight Doesn't Matter But Your Food Habits Do

MATTHIAS STUBER

Contents

10

INTRODUCTION

"Being healthy is not the outcome of a diet; it's the result of a lifestyle."

Hi. My name is Matthias Stuber, I am professional chef and certified nutritionist, worked for luxury brands like The Ritz-Carlton and Kempinski, that quote above? That's mine.

I firmly believe that diets are not the answer to losing weight and my belief comes from my own personal journey, which you can read about on my blog, Wander Culinaire.

There is no doubt about it – putting weight on is far easier for some people than losing it, and when they do lose it, it's even harder to keep it off. Sadly, most research on diets and their long-term effects show that most dieters will regain all their lost weight within a couple of years; in many cases, they'll have put even more on, leading to a vicious cycle of never-ending diets that simply don't work.

Most of us have been on several diets; when the first one doesn't work, we try another, and we keep on trying until we find one that works for us – that rarely, if ever, happens. For so long, we've had it drilled into us that diet and exercise are the only way to lose weight and keep it off, but that simply isn't true – at least not diets in the commercial sense of the word.

Even if you aren't on an "official" diet, you might be engaging in certain behaviors that make it seem like you are dieting. This is because such behaviors have been normalized by the diet industry, even encouraged, with no regard for the dangers over the long term. The longer you go on, the harder it becomes to determine just what "normal" is in terms of food.

Some of the ways you may be exhibiting dieting behaviors are:

- Constantly weighing yourself, sometimes several times a day
- Counting points, servings, or macros
- Exercising hard to try to burn off the food you just ate
- Basing your food choices purely on nutritional value
- Only eating low-fat, so-called "healthier" versions of meals
- Getting back on track by detoxing or cleansing

Diets and dieting are two completely different things. An actual diet is formal and has a ton of rules that you must follow to determine what you eat, how, and when. Dieting is less formal and has fewer rules, but you still beat yourself up when falling off the wagon, which is inevitable when you restrict what you can and can't eat.

None of this works, and both can lead to restrictive thoughts and behaviors, guilt, shame, stress, and anxiety, and can even lead to health disorders later in life.

That was the main reason why I started my own blog and YouTube Channel and am now publishing this book. To help people, like you, which are in the same situation I was, and managed to escape.

You see, it isn't only about what you eat. It's more about your relationship to food, how you eat and making small changes to your lifestyle that add up to a huge achievement. Not only can you lose excess weight easily, but you will also feel healthier and happier than ever. Which is for me more important at the first stage, than weight loss. For example: You don't like to do something, you are more likely to discontinue it, correct?

This book will walk you through these lifestyle changes and tell how each one will benefit you without throwing good money after bad on fad diets that simply don't work.

All this comes from the heart, my personal experience, and what I learned throughout my life, travels, and studies. Don't just take my word for it, though. Read on and find out how you can improve your life.

CHAPTER 1: WHY DIETS DO NOT WORK

How many times have you started a diet and failed miserably? Why did you start it? Today's society is cruel; we live in a world, especially social media world, where thin women and muscular men are put on pedestals and shown off as the way we should all look. The underlying message is this – if you are a thin woman or a muscular man, you have bags of confidence, you're healthy, and you achieve everything you set out to do. You are successful!

Anyone who doesn't conform to these looks is lazy, unhealthy, and a failure!

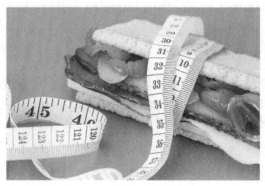

rawpixel

If that wasn't cruel enough, the diet industry has jumped on the bandwagon, trying to make us all believe that we need to be thinner if we want to be worthy. The more they make you feel bad about your appearance, the more likely you will throw money at one diet fad after another. And every one of those diets will fail, sooner or later.

That's why the diet industry is so profitable, a multi-billion-dollar industry that makes money hand over fist from diets that don't work. And all of this on your back! Let's face it; if you fail at one, you are more likely to choose one of the hundreds of other diets – and you'll keep trying, hoping one of them might just work.

Regardless, try to see it positive, as I believe that failure is part of the process, part of our development and personality.

Failure is a wonderful teacher. It is the only way to learn! Failure is a part of the process to become successful.

STEVE HARVEY, AMERICAN TELEVISION HOST

But changing your body, your well-being, your mindset is more than following a diet. It's a process of accepting the status quo in the first stage, shifting your mindset, and working on it. Sometimes in smaller steps, sometimes in larger steps, you keep going. But the most important part: it needs to become a habit, a culture, a lifestyle.

Your NEW LIFESTYLE!

Yes agree, it is work! You will not get it as a gift before you didn't do anything for it. You will get it as a gift after hard mental and physical work. And you will appreciate it even more and LOVE IT! Believe me!

The most important part: you need to start it! Better now, then never!

And with owning and reading this book you already did the first step. Which differentiates you from many others, which are only thinking about a change, but never starting it off!

Use this momentum to define your goals, whether it's losing

weight or just having a healthier nutrition which will make you more efficient from now onwards. Write these goals down, maybe create even a vision board of it. There are many ways of picturizing your upcoming success. But the most important part is, have your goals visible on a frequently used place or item. For example, on your office desk in a frame, on your home screen of your mobile device.

The second step record your status quo, like weight, pictures of yourself, when you started your lifestyle changing steps. This shall track your positive process and motivate you even more! Motivation comes after starting something of, it will be not there at the beginning, believe me!

Will everything be perfect from day one? No, I can tell you. But the most important part… you started! And you will improve day by day from then on and weight loss will be the byproduct of your lifestyle change! So, weight loss should not be your primary goal, it will happen by itself. Magically! Like an autopilot!

But let me explain you first how everything began a few years back with me. I started off my journey of changing my lifestyle, with a critical moment, after my doctor presented shocking blood results to me. My cholesterol was spike high, he wanted to put me on a strict diet and give me medication. The standard procedure, I guess, in a time, where the pharma industry has a strong lobby, also in Germany.

Additionally, he made me very much aware of a potential heart attack if his suggestions would further be ignored. So, I made my research, in books, YouTube, online classes and so on. One year, a few books about nutrition, intermediate fasting, and being a certified nutritionist later, I changed my nutrition completely wherever I could. Till today I start eating at noon and stop eating at 8 pm. Drinking mainly enough water during the day and avoid refined sugar wherever I can. And guess what, my blood results are totally normal, without any medication and diets, only with a change of my nutrition, my lifestyle and self-awareness.

But talking about the diets and the financial costs of these, this is only the tip of the iceberg. There's much more to it than money.

There is plenty of research to show that when we start a diet, the weight loss is short-term, as it's mostly water weight at the beginning. Very little research shows you what happens to your weight further down the line – six months, a year, five years. They don't show you that most people regain every pound they lost on a diet and more. Those studies that have looked at this all show the same thing – your weight will always go back to how it was before you started the diet.

But that's not all.

Metabolism begins to slow, which is one of the worst things that could happen to those trying to lose or maintain their current weight. Even worse, your satisfaction with your appearance decreases, sending you into a vicious cycle of eating crap to feel better, dieting to lose weight, and then eating more crap when the diet fails.

Yo-yo dieting is physically harmful, more so than being a little overweight in the first place, and it's mentally and emotionally harmful, too.

The thing is it really isn't your fault. When you feel like you've failed at the latest diet, the blame should be placed squarely on the shoulders of the diet industry. They make us feel bad about not conforming to unrealistic expectations, and they charge the earth for diet plans that do not work, miracle cures that simply don't exist.

When we start a diet and restrict what we eat, the detrimental effects on our bodies are immediate. Our bodies need energy to function properly, which takes about 70% of our daily energy requirements. That includes proper functioning of the heart, lungs, kidneys, brain, and blood circulation – and that's just when we are asleep.

The human body works hard all the time, which takes serious energy. But that's not all. The body also needs energy to digest food and absorb it, for the immune system to

protect our bodies, for our cells to repair themselves, for our bodies to grow, to produce hormones, and so on. That's before the energy we need to go about our daily lives.

If you restrict your food intake, your body doesn't have enough fuel to do all these things. When there isn't enough to go around, the body begins to prioritize where the available energy should go and which functions it can slow down or stop to save energy, and that's when we start to feel the physical effects.

That's why so many people feel ill when they diet, with some of the more common experiences being:

- Fatigue
- Tiredness and lethargy
- Reduced sex drive
- Irregular menstruation
- Poor quality hair, skin, and nails
- Constantly feeling cold

These things happen because our bodies are working hard to conserve what energy it receives to keep vital functions going.

What would happen if we carried on restricting our intake? Or if we started heavy exercise, forcing our bodies to expend even more energy they don't have?

Our energy stores would begin to break down, and while that can include fat stores, it also means our muscles break down. Muscle is the one thing we don't want to lose because there is a close relationship between muscle and metabolism; less muscle equals a slower metabolism, which means food is converted to energy more slowly. The slower your metabolism, the more likely you will gain weight and struggle to lose it.

All this leads to the body putting in even more work to conserve energy, which will begin to slow things down. That includes:

- Heart rate slowing down
- Blood pressure falling
- A slower digestive system leading to bloating, constipation, and abdominal discomfort
- A slower metabolism
- A slower brain which means poor concentration, poor thinking skills, and an inability to solve problems

Not looking good, is it?

FOOD DEPRIVATION

What if you're not bothered about how dieting affects you physically? Have you considered the way these diets affect your food relationship? How often have you started a diet that seems to work, but then you put a foot wrong and eat something you shouldn't? Many people find that restrictive diets leave them constantly hungry, leading to them foraging in the cupboards for whatever they can find to eat, whether it's on their diet plan or not. Then they beat themselves up, label themselves greedy, or say they don't have the willpower to stick to the diet. That's not true. Restrictive diets lead to one thing, and one thing only – deprivation.

Deprivation may be psychological or physical. When you restrict your food intake consistently, you force your body into a negative energy balance, making it scream for more energy. Food is a requirement – it fuels our bodies and helps us survive. When our body doesn't have enough energy to do what it needs, it will drive us to eat something so that it can do its work. That's why diets often leave us hungry and can lead to uncontrolled eating, leading to guilt – a vicious cycle we struggle to get out of.

Deprivation isn't just about overall restriction. It can also be when you restrict specific kinds of food. Think about it – how many times have you told yourself you will never eat cookies, candy, or chips again? You might resist the temptation at first, but your cravings get the better of you, and before you know it, you've eaten a family-sized bag of candy – by yourself! That's deprivation for you. You may eat enough food throughout the day, but by depriving yourself of foods you really want, you place those foods on a pedestal in your mind – that makes them seem special and powerful.

We must stop making certain foods taboo and depriving ourselves of them. We need to start making peace with food again, rebuilding our relationship with it, and allowing ourselves to eat them again, but only as part of a balanced diet.

Deprivation can also lead to something known as "last supper eating." Let's say you decide cookies are not allowed. When some people give in and eat one, they leave it at that. Others believe that, as they've eaten one, they've failed, so they may as well eat the entire box. You might even decide that you need to eat all the cookies in the house, so there aren't any to tempt you tomorrow! This would not happen if you didn't ban cookies in the first place!

Another form of deprivation is when we stop our bodies from being their natural shape and weight. Our height is already predetermined when we are born, but so is our natural weight range. This is known as a set point range, and although our environment has some influence over it, for example, poor nutrition, or neglect, the biggest influencer is genetics. Simply put, our predetermined weight range is set and not intended to be changed.

If we start a diet and lose some weight, our bodies go to work on trying to regulate the weight and get it back to that set point. How? By sending out hunger signals, making us think more about food, obsessing over it, and even slowing our metabolism. Our bodies push even harder when we ignore all this, which can lead to out-of-control eating. It's quite simple – genetics play a huge part in our weight, and there is nothing we can do to change our set point range.

If we want a good relationship with our bodies and food, we need to accept the body we have. We need to stop depriving ourselves of certain foods and ensure we feed our bodies the nutrition needed for healthy, effective functioning.

DIETING LEADS TO BINGING

Most dieters will tell you that their diets often end in binge eating, often saying that they fell into a period of "out-of-control" eating. Yet many of them will never see the diet as being to blame; instead, that blame lands on them and an apparent lack of willpower.

What they don't seem to be able to grasp is that willpower plays no part in it – it's the diet and the restrictions it imposes that cause people to binge on food. By their very nature, diets are restrictive and full of so-called "forbidden" foods. Studies have shown these restrictions to:

- Make "forbidden" foods more desirable
- Increase the reward stimulation, which means dieters who eat "forbidden" foods get higher rewards and more pleasure from eating them than someone not on a diet
- Make people crave sugar and fat, which leads to binge eating
- Make the brain come alive when these foods are about, increasing cravings and binge eating

So, it really shouldn't surprise anyone that they can't stop eating these "forbidden" foods when they fall off their diet.

Falling off a diet in this way also leads to something known as the "Last Supper Syndrome," which is when you tell yourself this is your last binge; you'll get back on your diet tomorrow, and these foods will never pass your lips again – until the next time.

That mentality, fueled by the diet industry, leads to the diet-binge-diet cycle:

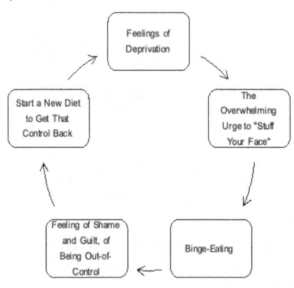

I'm pretty sure most of us have experienced this cycle more than once in our lives. However, there is a light at the end of the tunnel – a way out of the cycle.

First, allow yourself to eat anything – nothing is considered "forbidden." When you give yourself this permission, you begin to experience something called "food habitation," which decreases the high appeal of some foods.

What is Food Habituation?

Habituation is when we can adapt to an experience and, as we repeat that experience, we get less pleasure from it, which applies to "forbidden" foods. When you know that you can eat anything you want at any time and enjoy them repeatedly, their novelty will soon disappear, and you won't need to eat so much of them, thus reducing the chances of binging.

However, this can only happen when no foods are disallowed.

When you go on a diet, and certain foods are not allowed, you will never tire of binging on those foods – you know you will start your diet again tomorrow, after all!

When you allow yourself to eat anything, whenever you want, your attitude towards food changes; you begin to think of food differently, less of an "I know this food is forbidden" and more of a "do I really WANT this food right now?" attitude. As time passes, you begin to enjoy everything and automatically eat less because you know you can have it whenever you want – nothing is restricted! That eliminates the need to overeat.

However, as you will find later in the book, there are some foods you should "forbid" yourself from eating, not because you are on a diet but because of the serious health issues they cause.

Here's where you can face down the diet industry and beat them at their own game. We know diets don't work, and the best way you can beat the industry is to do the following:

1. **Allow Yourself to Eat**

Let yourself enjoy all foods; don't feel guilty when you eat candy or ice cream. That way, you give all foods the same emotional equivalence and the urgency to eat bad foods disappears.

2. **Ask Yourself What You Truly Want**

When you allow yourself to eat anything, you can begin to consider what you want. You may not want that cookie because it doesn't hold the same appeal as it did when it was forbidden.

3. **Tune in to Your Feelings**

When you decide you want to eat something, take a minute to notice it. Be mindful in your eating – notice how the food tastes and what it feels like. More importantly, notice how it makes you feel. Does it give you pleasure? Does it taste better now you have permission to eat it whenever you want? If you decide you aren't enjoying it, stop eating. Do this with everything, and you will soon stop eating those foods you no longer enjoy, foods you used to salivate over because they were forbidden.

4. **Wave Goodbye to Your Inner Critic**

Whenever you begin to tell yourself you are eating "bad" food, criticize yourself or make deals with the devil – if I eat this chocolate now, I'll go on a strict diet for the next month – you are making rules that lead to restrictive eating. Restriction leads to deprivation which leads to overeating and binging. Instead, you need to make eating into something you get satisfaction from – if you want a piece of chocolate, have it. You are not a bad person.

Diets tend to focus our attention on the wrong things – they make us believe that we need to have a specific body shape and be a specific weight if we are to be happy and successful. Diets remove our natural ability to think about anything other than food, stopping us from directing energy and attention to everything else that matters to us in our lives.

When you allow a diet to take priority, it can affect your family, friendships, career, and hobbies. You begin to feel unhappy and look for ways to make yourself feel better – another diet, perhaps. You need to be clear on your goal – what do you think a new diet will fix? Then ask yourself another question – can you fix this without suffering the negatives of dieting?

Focus your attention back on happiness, connections to others, and pride, and you'll feel healthier and better than you ever did on a diet – that's what you want to achieve, isn't it?

Now you know why diets don't work, the rest of this book will look at simple changes you can make to your lifestyle to repair your relationship with food and make yourself feel 100% healthier and happier.

CHAPTER 2: DITCH THE SUGAR

I try my hardest to avoid refined sugar in my life, and there's a good reason for it. In my recipes later in this book, you'll notice that I use alternatives – refined sugar has no place in my food!

Sugar isn't just for sweetening your tea or coffee, and it has many different names, including glucose, fructose, sucrose, and corn syrup, to name just a few. However, regardless of the name they go by, all sugars are carbohydrates, and they all give us energy.

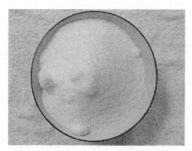

Wikimedia

We mostly associate sugar with fizzy sodas, baked goods, candy, and cookies, but almost all food has sugar. It's hard to control sugar consumption because it's often added to foods we wouldn't think of, which is why checking labels is so important. The RDA (recommended daily allowance) is no more than 11 grams of sugar per day or 5% of your calorie intake. The WHO maintains that we should never exceed 25 grams of sugar daily, but it might shock you to realize that we all eat far more than that. Let's look at the top 10 sugar-eating countries in the world just to give you an idea of how much we eat:

1. **USA** - 126 grams daily – ¼ of a pound of sugar per day!
2. **Germany** – 103 grams daily
3. **Netherlands** – 102 grams daily
4. **Ireland** – 97 grams daily
5. **Australia** – 96 grams daily
6. **Belgium** – 95 grams daily
7. **UK** – 93 grams daily
8. **Mexico** – 92 grams daily
9. **Finland** – 91 grams daily
10. **Canada** – 89 grams daily

These are average figures, but, as you can see, they are way above the RDA, making it easy to see why obesity is fast becoming a major health issue.

THE SIDE EFFECTS OF REFINED SUGAR

Refined sugar is made from sugar beets or sugar cane, and the plants are processed to get the sugar. Refined sugar is normally in the form of sucrose, a combination of fructose and glucose. Our bodies break it down quickly when we consume it, causing our blood sugar and insulin levels to shoot up. You may have noticed that when you eat something that contains refined sugar, you don't really feel full. That's because the body digests refined sugar very quickly, regardless of the number of calories consumed. By contrast, the natural sugar found in fruit is not digested so quickly, as fruit contains fiber which slows metabolism and expands in your gut, making you feel fuller for longer.

Eating refined sugar can lead to several health issues, including type 2 diabetes, obesity, heart disease, dementia, depression, liver disease, and some cancers.

These are all things we should take note of – the more sugar we eat, the higher our risk of serious disease. A couple of years ago, I decided to try an experiment. It was 2019, the start of a new year, and I had just qualified as a nutritionist. I wanted to change my life, so I opted to ditch refined sugar.

First, I removed everything from my kitchen cupboards that contained sugar, including hidden sugars. I checked the labels on everything, ditched all sorts of foods, and replaced them with foods that didn't have sugar. What happened?

Well, on the first day without sugar, I tried a raw carrot. It didn't taste great; I'm a professional chef, and I was really disappointed in its flavor. I put the rest of the carrots in the chiller, thinking I would try again in a few days.

The first few days without sugar, I felt really bad. My sugar cravings were bad, even waking me at night. I had terrible mood swings and headaches, and I just felt tired. Now I know that these were my body screaming at me for sugar. This continued for several days until my body had adjusted to not having sugar. On the sixth day, I tried a raw carrot again, and the flavor was amazing – it tasted sweet and carroty! I didn't feel so tired, and my thoughts were clear – I was stunned! From then on, I vowed to educate myself and others about the importance of nutrition and how it affects us every day – that's why I wrote my blog and produced a YouTube channel full of my healthy, tasty recipes.

SUGAR ALTERNATIVES

So, what can you use instead of sugar? Well, there are tons of sugar alternatives, but I use the following in my recipes:

- **Maple Syrup:** - packed with minerals and antioxidants, maple syrup is made by concentrating the sugar maple sap from maple trees. Make sure you only use natural maple syrup; there are tons of fakes out there.

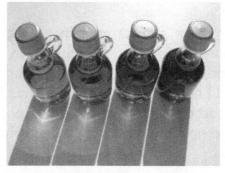

Wikimedia

- **Date Paste:** dates are full of vitamins, minerals, and fiber, so substituting sugar with date paste not only eliminates the risks of refined sugar, but it also adds more nutrients and finer to your food. Date paste is made by blending dates with water and can also be used instead of honey, although it isn't as sweet.

- **Natural Honey:** honey has more nutrients than refined sugar and contains vitamins, minerals, and antioxidants. It is good for the gut and easier to digest but make sure it is natural honey – some manufacturers add glucose syrup, which is no better than sugar.

- **Coconut Sugar:** Coconut sugar is never refined, meaning it retains its minerals and vitamins and never causes blood sugar levels to spike and drop. It is plant-based, a natural sweetener like Stevia, and also contains natural fats that help mitigate the risks of heart diseases and high cholesterol. Coconut sugar also has inulin, a dietary fiber that improves gut health, balances blood sugar, and helps prevent colon cancer.

- **Agave Nectar:** Agave nectar doesn't provide as many nutrients as honey but has more than refined sugar. You don't need to use much as it is full of flavor and is commercially produced from the Agave species of plants.

There are loads more alternatives, including many different artificial sweeteners. However, the clue is in the name there – artificial – and, while some are okay, those that contain aspartame should be avoided. Aspartame has been linked to a higher risk of heart disease, type 2 diabetes, non-alcoholic fatty liver disease, and hormone-related cancers when consumed in large amounts.

All the alternatives I listed above are perfectly safe to use and can be found in almost any grocery store, no matter where you are.

HOW TO CUT YOUR SUGAR CONSUMPTION

We've been eating sugar for so long that cutting it out of our diets isn't going to be easy. Below, you can find a number of ways that can help you cut back, with a view to eliminating it from your diet altogether:

1. **Drink Fewer Sodas**

In most Western diets, especially in the USA, most of our added sugar comes from sodas, energy drinks, sports drinks, sweetened teas, and all sorts of other drinks. Even fruit juices and commercial smoothies can be packed with sugar. You might be interested to learn that your body won't treat the calories from these drinks the same way they treat food calories. Drink calories are "empty" calories – your body absorbs them quickly, rapidly pushing your blood sugar up and giving you no nutritional value.

Drinks don't fill you up like food does; people who drink a lot of sugary drinks don't compensate for the extra calories by eating less.

Cutting these out of your diet can help you lose weight and make you feel better overall. Some alternatives include:

- Water

- Herb teas

- Green or black tea

- Sugar-free carbonated water

- Black coffee

As you'll see in another chapter, water is the best, but if you can't drink it plain, add some slices of lemon, lime, or cucumber.

2. **Cut Out Sugary Dessert**

Dessert doesn't offer much nutritional value because most are packed with refined sugar, leaving you hungry and tired as your blood sugar spikes and falls. All they do is make you want even more sugar, and you might be shocked to learn that dairy and grain-based desserts, like donuts, pies, cakes, cookies, and ice cream, make up nearly 20% of the added sugar in the US diet.

There are plenty of healthier alternatives that can easily satisfy a sweet tooth, such as:

- Fresh fruit

- Baked fruit with a little fresh cream

- Greek yogurt with fruit or spices like cinnamon

- Dark chocolate – must be at least 70% cocoa

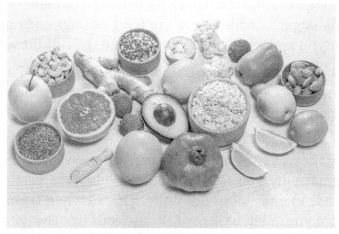

When you ditch sugary desserts for fresh fruit, you not only decrease the amount of refined sugar you consume but also eat more fiber, minerals, vitamins, and antioxidants.

3. Ditch Sugary Sauces

BBQ sauce, ketchup, sweet chili sauce, spaghetti sauce, and many other common sauces are found in kitchens worldwide. However, do you know how much sugar they contain? One tablespoon or 17 grams of ketchup has a whole teaspoon or 5 grams of sugar, meaning ketchup is nearly 30% sugar – that's more than ice cream!

Find sauces labeled "no added sugar" or use other ways to season your food, such as herbs, spices, mustard, chili, vinegar, mayonnaise, pesto, lime juice, or lemon juice.

4. Eat More Fat

Low-fat foods are unhealthy and buying low-fat versions of your favorite foods isn't doing you any favors. Too many people believe that fat is bad, but not all fat can be treated equally. Fat equals flavor, and when the fat is removed from the food to make it "healthier," that flavor has to be put back somehow – that's where the sugar is added, and the food usually ends up being worse for you and with more calories than the full-fat version.

Take a 6 oz serving of yogurt, for example. A low-fat vanilla version has 144 calories and 24 grams of sugar, while a full-fat plain version contains just 104 calories and 8 grams of sugar, naturally occurring in the milk.

We know that a high sugar intake can cause weight gain, which goes against why you would choose the low-fat version. This tells us that low-fat foods are unhealthy, so when trying to cut sugar from your diet, look for full-fat foods but always read the ingredients label, so you know exactly what you are eating.

5. Eat Clean, Whole Foods

When you eat a whole-food diet, you eat food that hasn't been refined or processed and doesn't contain additives or anything else artificial. This means eating whole fruit, whole grains, legumes, vegetables, meat on the bone, and whole fish. By contrast, ultra-processed foods are prepared or processed and contain a ton of sugar, salt, bad fats, and additives, all combined to make you think they taste wonderful – just another ploy to make you want to eat them. These foods include sugary cereals, soft drinks, fast foods, and chips.

In the American diet, about 90% of the added sugar comes from these foods, whereas when you prepare your meals using only whole foods, that figure drops to 8.7%. So, where you can, cook from scratch to avoid these sugars. You don't have to spend hours cooking elaborate, complicated meals in the kitchen. Simple meals can be the most delicious, as you'll see when you try my recipes.

6. Check Sugar Levels in Canned Foods

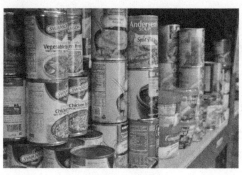

Flickr.com

While canned foods can be cheap and quick additions to your diet, most contain high sugar levels. Vegetables and fruits are full of naturally occurring sugars that don't cause your blood sugar to spike, but you should avoid foods canned in syrup or that list sugar on the ingredient label. Fruit is already sweet, so if you must buy canned, go for those labeled "no added sugar" or "packed in water." If you do buy canned foods with added sugar, it's a good idea to drain and rinse them before cooking and eating. That way, you can remove some of the sugar.

7. Watch Those So-Called "Healthy" Processed Snacks

Some snack foods may look healthy when you first look at them, especially when the words "natural" or "wholesome" are used to market them. These include protein bars, granola bars, and dried fruits, but it might surprise you to learn that there is just as much sugar in these foods as there is in candy bars. A good example is dried fruit. You might think it's really healthy because it contains high levels of antioxidants, fiber, and nutrients. However, it also has natural sugars in concentrated amounts, while some may even have been candied, which adds more sugar. While you shouldn't avoid eating dried fruits, you should be careful how much you consume.

Healthy alternative snacks include:

- Jerky – no added sugar
- Nuts
- Seeds
- Fresh fruit
- Boiled eggs

However, if you choose nuts or seeds, ensure they are raw, as roasted buts have often been coated in sugar.

8. Cut Down on Sugary Breakfast Cereal

Some cereals are packed with sugar, and some of the more popular ones contain an amount of added sugar that is more than half the weight of the cereal. One report found that one particular cereal has more than 50 grams of sugar per serving – that's 12 teaspoons! Would you put 12 teaspoons of sugar in a bowl and eat it?

That same report showed granola, a so-called healthy food, contains more sugar than any other cereal type. Other popular foods eaten for breakfast, such as waffles, pancakes, jams, and muffins, also contain a lot of extra sugar.

Cut these foods out and replace them with things like the following:

- Oatmeal with fresh fruit added
- Greek yogurt with nuts and fruit
- Avocado toast
- Egg scramble with vegetables and cheese

All of these have less sugar and more protein and fiber, making you feel fuller for longer and eliminating the need for snacking between meals.

9. **Always Read Labels**

Cutting down on sugar isn't just about not eating sweet foods because it's already clear that many other foods, such as granola and sauces, contain it. Fortunately for all of us, food manufacturers must now disclose the addition of added sugars on food labels, and where food contains them, you will see them under total carbohydrates. In some cases, sugar will be listed as an ingredient, and as a rule of thumb, the higher in the ingredient list it is, the more there is of it.

However, you won't always see it as sugar because added sugars have more than 50 names. Some of the most common are:

- HFCS – high fructose corn syrup
- Cane sugar
- Cane juice
- Dextrose
- Maltose
- Rice syrup
- Invert sugar
- Molasses
- Caramel

You know your food has added sugars if you see any of these on the label.

10. **Eat More Protein**

Reports show that people who eat a lot of sugar tend to eat more food overall and gain more weight. Conversely, those who eat less sugar but a diet high in fiber and protein tend to lose weight more easily. Protein and fiber fill you up quickly, reducing hunger and cravings. That is especially true of protein and eating 25% more protein in your diet can reduce your sugar cravings by an incredible 60%.

To stop your cravings for sugar, eat whole fish, meat, eggs, avocados, full-fat dairy, and nuts.

11. Switch to Natural Sweeteners

The stores are full of artificial sweeteners that contain no sugar and no calories, like aspartame and sucralose. However, these have been linked to gut bacterial imbalances, which can cause blood sugar spikes, cravings, and weight gain. This is why you should avoid anything with the word "artificial" in it.

Instead, choose natural sweeteners, such as Stevia, Truvia, monk fruit, erythritol, allulose, honey, and so on. While some powdered sweeteners are processed, they are all derived from nature.

12. Get Rid of High Sugar Foods

If your cupboards are full of high-sugar foods, you will eat them; it's as simple as that. If you live alone, you can simply stop buying them, but it gets a bit harder when you live with others. So, if you must have sugar in the house, come up with a way of distracting yourself when you feel like a craving is coming on. Do a puzzle, go for a walk, anything that takes your mind off the sugar. Alternatively, stock up on low-sugar healthy snacks.

13. Get Enough Sleep

One of the most important factors in good health is sleep. It's no good getting 8 hours of sleep a night if it's poor quality because this has been linked to poor concentration, depression, a poor immune system, and obesity.

However, poor sleep or lack of sleep may also contribute to what you eat, and some studies show that people who don't sleep enough are more prone to eating foods higher in calories, sugar, salt, and bad fats. One study reported that people who went to their beds late at night and had less sleep ate more fast food, calories, and soda and didn't eat as many fresh fruits and vegetables as those who slept for longer.

And another recent study on post-menopausal women has shown that a high sugar intake was linked to insomnia and poor-quality sleep. So, if you are struggling with bad food choices and sugar cravings, the answer might lie partly in getting a good night's sleep.

CHAPTER 3: DRINK MORE WATER

We all know we should drink more water than we do, but how much should we drink and why? How does water benefit us?

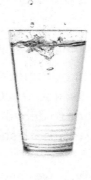

Rawpexel

THE BENEFITS
OF WATER

Let's start with the immense benefits that drinking water brings. First, the human body is roughly 60% water, so it makes perfect sense that we need water to help balance our body fluids – when you sweat or urinate, you lose water, which needs to be replaced. You should also be aware that human blood is 90% water, and every organ and cell need water for the human body to function properly.

Here are some of the main reasons why we need water:

- **Joint Lubrication:** our joints and spinal disks contain cartilage which is about 80% water. Not drinking enough water leads to dehydration which can decrease the joints' ability to absorb shock, resulting in pain and stiffness.
- **Mucus and Saliva:** we need saliva to help in the digestion process and to help keep our eyes, nose, and mouth moist, thus preventing damage from friction. Drinking water encourages saliva and mucus production and keeps the mouth clean; when you choose water over sugary drinks, you also lessen the risk of tooth decay and gum disease.
- **Oxygen Delivery:** as mentioned, blood is about 90% water and carries oxygen to where it is needed in the body. Dehydration slows this process.
- **Skin Health:** when you don't drink enough water, your skin can begin to wrinkle and age prematurely, dry out,

and you are at a higher risk of skin disorders.

- **Cushioning for Sensitive Tissues:** this includes the brain and the spinal cord. Dehydration affects the brain's structure and function and slows the production of important neurotransmitters and hormones. Long-term dehydration can affect your thinking and reasoning abilities.
- **Body Temperature Regulation:** some water is stored in the center layers of the skin, and when your body heats up, that water is eliminated as sweat. When the sweat evaporates, the body cools down. It has been suggested that dehydration can lead to an increase in body heat and an ability to tolerate heat strain. Should heat stress occurs, a dehydrated person would be less able to cope with it than a person who drinks enough water.
- **Proper Functioning of the Digestive System:** the digestive system requires water to function properly, particularly the bowels. Lack of water leads to too much acid in the stomach, constipation, and digestive issues, increasing the risk of stomach ulcers, heartburn, and acid reflux.
- **Waste Removal:** water is necessary to help the body sweat and remove feces and urine from the body.
- **Blood Pressure:** when you don't drink enough water, your blood can thicken, leading to high blood pressure.
- **It Helps Your Breathing:** when you don't drink enough water, your body restricts your airways to stop you from losing water. That makes allergies, asthma, and other breathing issues worse.
- **It Helps Make Nutrients and Mineral More Accessible:** nutrients and minerals dissolve in water, ensuring they get to the parts of the body where they are needed.
- **Prevents Damage to the Kidneys:** the kidneys are responsible for fluid regulation in the body, and not

drinking enough can lead to kidney damage, including kidney stones and disease.

- **Boosts Exercise Performance:** If you are dehydrated during exercise, it may lower your performance. One report showed that dehydration reduced performance in sports or exercise activities that lasted at least half an hour.
- **Weight Loss:** consuming water instead of soda and fruit juice can help you lose weight, especially if you drink a glass of water 30 minutes before each meal.
- **Reduces Hangovers:** if you drink alcohol, alternating each drink with a glass of unsweetened soda water loaded with lemon and ice can help prevent hangovers by reducing alcohol consumption.
- **Improves Focus:** dehydration causes the brain cells to shrink a little, resulting in a foggy feeling. Drinking more water throughout the day eliminates this, allowing you to concentrate better.

In terms of weight loss, water is better at helping keep your calories balanced than soda. Of course, a glass of water has far fewer calories than, say, a glass of cola, so your calorie intake drops by replacing that cola with water. However, you also benefit from less sugar, which lowers your risk of diabetes and heart disease. Too many people think that by replacing sugary sodas with fruit juices, they are being healthy, but this is wrong – fruit juice contains fructose, which is nothing more than a different form of sugar and still full of calories.

Pro Tip

Whenever you feel hungry, ask yourself a question – have I drunk enough today? Dehydration mimics hunger; more often than not, drinking a glass of water relieves hunger pangs. Try it – when you feel peckish, have a glass of water, and wait 20 minutes. The same applies to headaches – most are caused by dehydration, and a glass or two of water can often help relieve the symptoms.

FAQ

How should I drink my water? What's the best technique?

Start by purchasing a water bottle that holds 1 liter or 34 oz. Fill it with filtered water and have a swig as soon as you wake before you have your first coffee or brush your teeth. Take it with you everywhere and keep drinking it. Make sure you refill it at least once during the day – you are aiming to drink 2 liters (68 oz) per day as a minimum. If you can drink more, go for it but don't overdo it.

How Much Water is Considered Enough?

That depends on many things and will vary from person to person. However, as a minimum, aim for 2 liters (68 oz) per day. If you want to be precise, use the following formula to work out exactly how much you should be drinking:

Your body weight in pounds x 0.5

For example, if you weigh 200 lbs, your calculation would be:

200 x 0.5 = 100

That's how many ounces of water you need to drink per day.

Do I Have to Drink Plain Water?

Absolutely not but be careful how you flavor it. Adding a couple of slices of fresh lemon or cucumber is a nice way of flavoring water, and lemon comes with another benefit – it helps burn body fat and adds much-needed vitamins to your water.

One way of ensuring you drink water during the day is to drink one glass (8 oz.) of water around 15 to 30 minutes before every meal. This will fill you up, and you will eat far less, thus taking in fewer calories.

CHAPTER 4: TRY INTERMITTENT FASTING

As mentioned at the start, I follow an intermittent fasting lifestyle – it's fair to say that it's the only thing that has really worked for me, and done properly, it can result in huge benefits, not just in weight loss.

Generally, I have my first meal at noon and do not eat anything after 8 pm. The idea is to do all your eating within an 8-hour window and allow your body 16 hours to rest. This method worked and has helped me in so many ways.

Right now, intermittent fasting (IF) is one of the world's most popular weight loss and wellness methods undertaken by millions of people worldwide. Not only do people use it to lose weight, but they also use it to make themselves healthier and simplify their lifestyles. Many studies have been done on the effects of intermittent fasting, and they all agree that it can have a powerful, positive effect on your brain and body and even help prolong your life.

Let's take a quick look at this amazing method.

WHAT IS INTERMITTENT FASTING?

It is a pattern of eating that cycles between periods of eating and fasting. Rather than dictating what you eat as most diets do, intermittent fasting is based around when you should eat for maximum benefits. Therefore intermittent fasting is not described as a diet; rather, it is an eating pattern or a lifestyle.

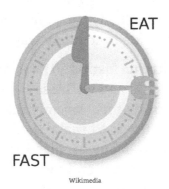

EAT

FAST

Wikimedia

Fasting has long been practiced. Centuries ago, hunter-gatherers didn't have access to refrigerators or grocery stores, and food wasn't available all year round. Much of the time, they had nothing to eat because there was no food available. This resulted in humans being able to function without eating for long periods. In fact, it is considered more natural to fast on occasion than it is to eat several meals per day.

Some people also fast for religious reasons, for example, Christianity, Buddhism, Judaism, and Islam.

INTERMITTENT FASTING METHODS

There is more than one way to do intermittent fasting; each method involves dividing the days or week into periods of eating and fasting. During fasting, little to no food is consumed.

The most popular methods of intermittent fasting are:

- **16/8:** also known as Lean gains, this is the most popular method. This is the method I choose to do, and it requires you to miss breakfast and to eat your meals within a set 8-hour period, i.e., 12 noon to 8 pm. The remaining 16 hours are for fasting.

- **Eat-Stop-Eat:** this method requires you to undertake a 24-hour fast one or two days per week. For example, after your final meal of the day, you do not consume any more food until the same meal the next day. Do this twice a week, but not on consecutive days, and eat normally on the remaining days of the week.

- **5:2:** this method allows you to eat normally for five days of the week and, on the other two days, you consume between 500 and 600 calories. Again, the two days should not be consecutive.

All of these methods reduce how many calories you eat in a given day or week, provided you eat sensibly. By this, I mean that during your eating window, or on days when you can eat normally, you eat a healthy, balanced diet. If you stuff your face with poor-quality, sugary, or processed foods, it won't work. You don't have to cut out things like chocolate altogether, though, as you'll see in my recipes later in the book – moderation is key!

HOW INTERMITTENT FASTING AFFECTS HORMONES AND CELLS

When you undertake a fasting period, many things begin to happen in your body on molecular and cellular levels.

For example, your hormone levels will begin to adjust, ensuring your stored body fat is more accessible and can be burned as energy. And your cells begin to repair themselves and regenerate. Some changes that fasting kickstarts in your body include:

- **Higher Levels of HGH:** HGH or human growth hormone levels shoot sky-high, increasing by as much as five times. This helps your body burn fat and helps your muscles grow, both of which result in weight loss.

- **Improvements to Insulin Sensitivity:** fasting lowers the risk of insulin sensitivity, and your body's insulin levels also drop significantly. This enables stored body fat to be easily accessible.

- **Cellular Repair:** when you fast, your cells begin to repair themselves but also digest dysfunctional old proteins, removing them from inside the cells.

- **Gene Expressions:** your genes change how they

function in terms of longevity and how they protect you against diseases.

All of these changes bring about the significant benefits of intermittent fasting.

WEIGHT LOSS

The first and most common benefit for people who start intermittent fasting is weight loss, which is the commonest reason people try it. Because you eat less food overall, IF results in a lower calorie intake and changes your hormone levels, thus promoting weight loss. As well as increasing growth hormone levels of growth hormones and reducing insulin levels, IF also increase the levels of noradrenaline released, a fat-burning hormone more commonly known as norepinephrine. These changes can lead to an increase in metabolic rate.

In 2014, one study determined that intermittent fasting can result in weight loss of 3% to 8% over 24 weeks, a significant percentage given the low rate of most diets. The same study also determined that people who followed an intermittent fasting lifestyle lost between 4% and 7% of their waist circumference, indicating that their belly fat had decreased significantly. Belly fat is one of the most dangerous as it settles around your organs and leads to many high-risk diseases. It has also been shown that IF causes far less muscle loss than other diets that restrict calories continually.

However, you do need to keep in mind that this can only happen if you consume fewer calories. You won't lose weight if you binge on huge amounts of food or eat crappy junk food during your eating window; it could even have the opposite effect.

HEALTH BENEFITS

Intermittent fasting has been studied in both humans and animals, and the studies don't just show the significant weight loss benefits; they also show that IF can have great benefits on your brain and body. The main benefits are:

- **Weight Loss:** as already mentioned, done properly, IF can help you lose belly fat and weight without going on a restrictive diet.

- **Insulin Resistance:** insulin resistance is reduced, blood sugar can drop by up to 6%, and fasting insulin levels can drop by up to 31%, all lowering your risk of type 2 diabetes.

- **Inflammation:** some studies have shown that IF can reduce inflammation markers, which are one of the biggest drivers of chronic disease.

- **Heart Health:** in some cases, IF can reduce LDL, or bad cholesterol, inflammatory markers, blood triglycerides, insulin resistance, and blood sugar, all huge risk factors for heart disease.

- **Cancer:** studies on animals have shown that IF can go some way to preventing cancer.

- **Brain Health:** IF increases BDNF, a brain hormone, and can help new nerve cells grow and protect against diseases like Alzheimer's.

- **Anti-Aging:** studies on rats showed that IF extended their lifespan by up to 83%.

Much of the research is still quite new; some studies were only short-term and only carried out on animals. However, the benefits are hard to deny, and I can testify to how much intermittent fasting has helped me not just to drop excess weight but improve my overall health and well-being.

A SIMPLER LIFESTYLE

It is pretty simple to start a healthy eating regime but incredibly hard to keep it going. Not only do we lose interest, but it's hard work to plan all those meals and cook them every day. That's where intermittent fasting comes in to make things easier. With IF, there's no need to plan intricate menus and meals, and, as you are not eating as much, there is less cooking and cleaning to do. This is why IF has become popular, as it simplifies life while improving your health – a win-win situation.

That said, not everyone can do intermittent fasting. Those who are already underweight, struggle to put weight on, or have had eating disorders in the past (or currently) should never attempt IF without prior consultation with their medical caregiver. In these cases, IF can be harmful without medical supervision.

Some studies say IF doesn't offer the same benefits for women as it does for men. Much of this comes down to hormonal fluctuations, particularly in women who are still ovulating. Some studies have also shown that IF reduced insulin sensitivity in men and worsened blood sugar control in women.

There are also reports of women whose monthly cycles stopped when they started an IF lifestyle but restarted when they gave it up. And animal studies have also shown that female rats became emaciated, infertile, and in some cases, masculinized; however, there are no human studies to back this up.

While there is nothing stopping women from following an IF lifestyle, they must ease into it gradually, carefully monitoring how their bodies react, and, should any problems arise, they must stop it immediately. If necessary, do it under strict medical supervision.

SAFETY AND SIDE EFFECTS

One of the main side effects of IF can be hunger, and when you first start, you may feel weaker than normal, and your brain may be a little sluggish. However, these effects are only temporary; once your body has adapted to your new way of eating, it will be fine.

Medical advice should be sought if you have a medical condition, especially important if:

- You have diabetes

- You have trouble regulating blood sugar

- You have low blood pressure

- You are on any prescribed or OTC medications

- You are underweight

- You struggle to put weight on

- You have had or still have an eating disorder

- You are trying to get pregnant

- You have or have had amenorrhea

- You are already pregnant or breastfeeding

That said, intermittent fasting has an incredible safety profile because, provided you are in good health and already well-nourished, not eating for a while is not dangerous.

FAQ

These are some of the commonly asked questions about intermittent fasting:

Can I Consume Liquids During My Fasting Days/Windows?

Yes. You can drink as much water as you want, herbal or fruit teas, black or green tea, natural fruit juices, and black coffee. You can have a little milk or cream but do not overdo it; do not add sugar to your drinks. Coffee is an excellent drink when fasting, as it has been shown to curb hunger pangs.

Isn't Skipping Breakfast Bad for You?

No. Many people who skip breakfast do not have a healthy lifestyle, but provided you eat a healthy balanced diet for the rest of the day, there is nothing wrong with missing breakfast.

Can I Take Supplements During My Fasting Periods?

Yes, but be aware that some supplements work better if you take them with food, such as fat-soluble vitamins.

Can I Work Out When in a Fasted State?

Yes. You could also consider taking BCAAs (branched-chain amino acids) before your workout – these are readily available online and in health stores.

Doesn't Fasting Result in Muscle Loss?

Every diet or weight loss method can result in muscle loss, which is why you should do some weightlifting and ensure you eat enough protein. That said, studies have shown that IF causes less muscle loss than traditional calorie-restricted diets.

Will My Metabolism Slow Down?

No. Studies have shown that fasting can actually speed up your metabolism if done for no more than 48 hours. However, longer fasts can suppress metabolism and cause you to gain weight or, at the very least, not lose any.

Can Children Fast?

It's not a great idea to allow kids to fast; they already have much faster metabolisms and need more food than adults.

GETTING STARTED

There's a good chance you've already fasted, probably many times. How often have you eaten your final meal of the day, gone to bed, woken late, and not eaten again until lunchtime? That is an example of 16:8 IF.

Some people do this instinctively because they aren't hungry in the morning.

16:8 is considered the easiest way to start an IF lifestyle, and it's much easier to maintain. If you stop eating at 8 PM and don't start again until noon the next day, most of your fasting time is taken up by sleeping – no effort at all!

If you get on well with this method and it makes you feel great, you can also increase things. Try moving on to a method where you fast for 24 hours once or twice a week or restrict your calories on two days of the week.

Another way to start is simply to fast when it works for you. If you don't feel hungry or you get home late from work and can't be bothered to cook, just skip a meal. You don't need to follow a structured plan, but some people prefer to do so, as it makes it easier to get into IF.

Don't be afraid to experiment; settle with something that works for you, provides the benefits you want, and that you enjoy.

Make sure that you eat a healthy, balanced diet and drink plenty of water during your eating days or window.

CHAPTER 5: CUT
SOME CARBS

We all know how much enjoyment we get from things like chips, candy, and cookies, but we also know that the thrill we get from eating them doesn't last long. That's because they are simple carbs – they are not good for you and result in you feeling bad for eating them.

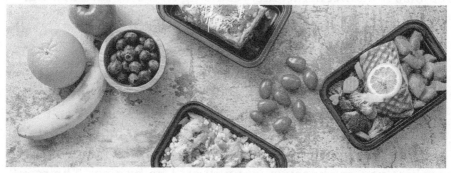
wellhub

It doesn't matter how bad these foods make us feel after we've eaten them; we can't seem to stop – we are addicted. And yes, many studies confirm that it IS an addiction. And it doesn't matter how careful you are about what you consume. One chocolate chip cookie contains as many calories as a whole bowl of oatmeal.

To be honest, carbs are everywhere and hard to turn your back on. So, what happens to your body if you do resist them?

Here are some of the benefits of cutting carbs from your diet:

1. **You start to burn fat**

Almost immediately. When you cut down on the number of carbs you eat, especially those dense in calories, you automatically cut down your calorie intake. Do this daily, forcing your body to turn to the fat stored in your belly and start burning that for energy instead of the glucose that comes from carbohydrates.

Tip:

Before you eat breakfast, do some exercise. Working out on an empty stomach forces your body to burn that belly fat instead of the food you ate first. If you can get hold of it, you can also drink a cup of Pu-erh tea, known to lower the blood's fat concentrations, resulting in faster fat burning.

2. **You don't feel so hungry**

That might sound weird; how can you be less hungry if you eat less food? Calories don't fill you up; protein, fiber, and healthy fats do. Simple carbs, like those cookies, don't have any of those three, so all they do is pump empty, harmful calories into your body. It doesn't matter how many of those cookies you eat because you will still be hungry. The result is that you are constantly hungry and sluggish all the time, making you more likely to head for something junky and sugary.

Tip:

Make your first meal of the day – no matter what time it is – one filled with high protein and fat. Try Greek yogurt, chia pudding, or an egg and vegetable scramble.

3. Your belly shrinks

When you trade simple carbs for foods high in fiber, your belly begins to flatten out. On average, Americans eat just 15 g of fiber per day; the recommended daily allowance is 25 to 38. The result is that the healthy microbes that live in our gut and keep us slimmer don't have a lot to eat, while the unhealthy ones that just love sugar do. Those unhealthy microbes make us bloat and give us fat bellies.

Tip:

Start by making simple, natural swaps. Ditch worthless, flabby white bread for whole or multi-grain, or chuck some beans in your stir-fries and tacos. If you feel peckish between meals, have a few raw nuts – they are one of the best sources of healthy fat and fiber, helping to fight inflammation and boost your digestion. However, nuts are high in calories, so don't eat too many.

4. Your risk of diabetes plummets

Simple carbs are simple sugars, and we all know these don't do you any favors, not just by making you gain weight but by causing all sorts of other health conditions. If you eat too many simple carbs, your pancreas will produce too much insulin, leading to type 2 diabetes and insulin resistance.

Tip:

Your body doesn't digest complex carbs as quickly as simple ones because they are rich in fiber. Swapping simple for complex carbohydrates means your blood sugar doesn't spike and cause insulin to be released. The steadier you can keep your blood sugar, the less insulin is released, which means our body tissues stay insulin sensitive, which is always a good thing. Cutting simple carbs means your risks of diabetes and other diseases reduce significantly.

5. Your muscles get stronger

Virtually everything is healthier than a simple carb, even ice cream, and burgers. That's because simple carbs don't have any protein required for building muscles and keeping your hair, skin, and nails healthy. When you up your protein intake, you feed your body what it needs for your muscles to grow and strengthen without needing to find more food for more calories.

Tip:

If you get hungry between meals, stop eating sugary, simple carbs and try eating something with more protein to give your body fuel and stabilize your energy.

6. You have more energy

Don't think that all carbs are bad; they are not. Your body requires a certain amount of carbohydrates to function, especially your muscles and brain. When you ditch simple carbs in favor of complex carbs, such as fruit, vegetables, oatmeal, whole-wheat bread, quinoa, brown rice, and other whole-grain foods, you provide your body with a steady level of energy with none of the spikes and dips you get with simple carbs. You won't need to turn to bad food to boost your energy, and you won't find yourself struggling through the day.

Tip:

To be safe, you should not cut your carbs below 50 grams daily, regardless of those diets that tell you to eat no more than 20 grams. If you drop below 50 grams, you will likely experience energy dips, but you can easily reach that amount with half a banana and a cup of oatmeal.

COMBINING INTERMITTENT FASTING WITH LOW CARB

Most people who go low carb end up trying intermittent fasting, and most who choose an IF lifestyle end up cutting their carbs. Why?

Is it just that the two lifestyles overlap?

Is it that when you come across, yet another lie perpetrated by the so-called experts, such as you need to eat at least 5 times daily to stop yourself from starving or that cutting carbs leads to heart disease, you start to question everything else you've been told?

It could be that, but the primary reason why low carb and intermittent fasting lifestyles are synergistic. When you do one, the other works better; it's as simple as that. When you do low carb, it's easier to fast; when you fast, it's easy to do low carb.

They are the perfect support system for one another, and instead of that dreaded vicious cycle, we have a virtuous one.

Fasting upregulates the fat-burning mitochondria in our bodies, which creates new mitochondria. This promotes fat adaptation and reduces our reliance on sweet, sugary foods. Fat adaptation is perfect for a low-carb lifestyle because you can burn body fat easily, significantly reducing sugar cravings. When you cut carbs, you burn fat better, resulting in more mitochondria being built, a requirement for periods of fasting – you see how it all works?

If you want a low-carb lifestyle to work, you have to cut carbs. If you want an intermittent fasting lifestyle to work, you have to fast. If something can make those easier to do, it's all good.

Here are the benefits of combing low carb and IF:

1. You'll burn more fat

A study published in 2013 compared two groups of people on an alternate day fasting schedule. One group was on a low-fat diet, and the other was on a low-carb diet. Both groups showed weight loss and improvements in their metabolic health markers. However, the most body fat was lost by the low-carb group.

More recently, a study on a low-carb group doing a 6-month fasting schedule showed that body fat dropped even more, lean mass remained lean, and there was a significant decrease in fasting insulin. However, this study did not have a control group, and the group was consuming 30% of their diet as carbohydrates. Quite possibly, if that were dropped even lower, the results would be even better.

2. You won't lose so much muscle

A common criticism about intermittent fasting is that it can cause muscle loss, which is valid in some cases. If you are not sufficiently fat-adapted, you will still have high glucose requirements when your body is in a fasted state, and your body may start breaking muscle tissue down to get the amino acids and convert them to glucose.

When you cut carbohydrates, your body goes into ketosis and starts producing ketones; these ketones reduce how much glucose you need, thus sparing your muscle tissue. Several studies have shown that quite a few body tissues can use ketones instead of glucose, even more so when you are in ketosis. It's no real surprise that the studies mentioned above found that when people undertook both IF and low carb, their weight loss was all from body fat being burned. And you can spare your muscles even further by doing a little weightlifting.

3. You won't worry about food

Low-carb diets work because you feel fuller for longer, thus reducing your calorie intake. In standard calorie-counting diets, you have to track everything you eat, with the expectation that you might lose a pound or two, but low-carbers eat only until they are full, and the weight drops off.

In fact, many low-carbers fast without even realizing they are doing it, mostly because they are not hungry and skip meals. Those on high carbohydrate diets often need nothing short of superhuman willpower to fast and are constantly hungry – when they do fast, all they can think about is food, which is pure torture and leads to overeating when they break the fast.

4. You won't get postprandial blood glucose spikes

When you fast for a day or two and eat a high-carb meal, your blood glucose will spike immediately. When you eat a low-carb meal after the same fast, it doesn't – why not?

Imagine someone who has been living a low-carb lifestyle for a long-term having to take a glucose tolerance test. Most will fail these tests because their metabolism is fat-based, and they cannot handle 75 grams of glucose. Their bodies are set for fat burning, and suddenly they throw a load of sugar at it! That is not easy to do, and even those on a high-carb diet will likely fail, even if they are in tip-top health.

When you come out of a fast, your body is burning fat, and while you don't have the same level of glucose intolerance as a low-carber, your energy comes from fat, which raises the risk of postprandial blood sugar spikes.

If you want some carbs when you end a fast, you should break it with a session of hard exercise and then consume those carbs. The exercise clears the glycogen out of your system, simulating glucose intolerance and giving the carbohydrates a storage space.

Or you could just adopt a low-carb lifestyle and avoid the issue in the first place.

5. You won't overdo the re-feeds

Fasting is excellent for reducing your calorie intake and inducing weight loss. That's why IF works by creating a boundary of sorts to help us control what we eat and how often. However, when they break their fast, some people overeat on their re-feed. They've been without food all day and are starving, so they pig out and eat far too many calories, often from the wrong sorts of food. That negates all the good the fast did.

If you are following a low-carb lifestyle, you won't do this. The risk of overeating is lower because the right low-carb foods are filling, and you won't turn to junk food because low-carb diets eliminate junk food.

6. Your insulin levels will normalize

When your insulin levels are high, you store fat, typically in adipose tissue, which makes fat-burning very hard. A chronic level of insulin, or hyperinsulinemia, significantly raises the risk of Alzheimer's disease and cancer and has also been linked to atherosclerosis.

IF is a great way of reversing hyperinsulinemia. Recent studies show that alternate day fasting brought about similar body weight reductions but also significantly improved insulin and insulin resistance better than regular calorie restrictions. Low-carb eating also reverses hyperinsulinemia because cutting out the bad carbs reduces insulin levels.

Insulin does have its place in the body, and we couldn't live without it. However, too much of it at the wrong time and for prolonged periods leads to serious health risks, but you can normalize your levels by combining IF and low-carb.

So, let's clear this up – if you are not following a low-carb lifestyle, should you avoid intermittent fasting?

Not really.

You can fast while eating a high-carb diet, provided you include exercise, specifically weightlifting, in your regime. One of the best ways to do it is to eat a low-fat, high-carb diet on training days, ensuring your exercise is done at or close to the end of the fast. On your non-training days, eat high-fat, low-carb meals. This method significantly increases insulin sensitivity and provides storage space for the carbs you consume.

BULLETPROOF COFFEE

Bulletproof coffee is a mainstay for many low-carbers and those on intermittent fasting. I said earlier that I follow the 16:8 method – I start my eating window at noon and end it at 8 pm. During that time, I not only eat balanced, healthy meals, but I also drink a lot of water.

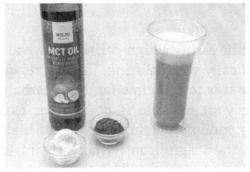

Flickr.com

However, some time ago, I wanted more energy first thing in the morning, so I tried drinking Bulletproof coffee. Invented by Dave Asprey, Bulletproof coffee has long been used in low-carb lifestyles to boost fat levels and weight loss while still being able to drink coffee.

So, what is it?

- **Coffee:** in sensible levels, caffeine helps keep you awake and full of energy, but it also helps burn fat and kickstarts your metabolism, as well as being full of antioxidants.

- **Butter:** not many people think of stirring butter into their coffee, but it gives the drink a creamy consistency, helps fill you up, provides energy, and also has lots of essential vitamins, such as Omega-3, vitamin A, and CLA, a fatty acid otherwise known as conjugated linoleic acid. If you've been following a low-carb lifestyle, you'll know that butter will burn fat.

- **MCT Coconut Oil:** medium-chain triglycerides, or MCT, helps you sustain your energy. Different fats have different jobs, allowing the brain and body to burn fat, not glucose.

- **Collagen Peptides** are excellent for muscle mass, heart health, bones, and skin.

And here's the recipe:

Bulletproof Coffee

Prep Time: 2 minutes

Cooking Time: 5 minutes

Total Time: 7 minutes

Serves 1

Equipment:

- Blender or hand blender

Ingredients:

- A mug of brewed coffee
- 10 g MCT coconut oil
- 10 g unsalted butter
- 10 g collagen peptides powder

Instructions:

1. Make your coffee as usual

2. Add it to your blender with all the other ingredients and blend for 10 seconds or until combined

It is your choice whether you choose to follow a low-carb lifestyle, but at the very least, I urge you to try intermittent fasting. It's worked for me, and you can try my recipes, all created by me, that you'll find at the end of this book.

CHAPTER 6: EAT SOME BRAINFOOD

Your brain is an important factor in your overall health and wellness. It's your body's control center; it keeps your lungs breathing, your heart beating, and your blood circulating, and it allows you to think, feel, and move.

That's why you need to keep it in good shape. What you eat plays an important part in the health of your brain and can also boost certain brain tasks, such as improving your concentration, focus, and memory.

11 foods you absolutely should include in your diet are listed below:

1. Fatty Fish

Most people know fatty fish is one of the best brain foods. This includes trout, salmon, albacore tuna, sardines, and herring, all rich in omega-3 fatty acids essential to brain health.

The human brain is 60% fat, and about half of that includes omega-3, used by the brain to build nerve and brain cells. Omega-3 is essential for memory and learning skills and offers other brain benefits.

It can help slow down mental decline relate to age and can help lessen the risks of diseases such as Alzheimer's. |Too little omega-3 can result in depression and risk of learning impairment.

Some studies have suggested that those who make fish a regular part of their diet have more gray matter, which is where most of the nerve cells responsible for emotion, memory, and decision-making live.

Including fatty fish in your diet is one of the best decisions you could ever make to keep your brain healthy.

2. Coffee

If you love a cup of coffee first thing when you wake, you'll be happy to learn that coffee is good for you – in moderation.

Two primary components in coffee support brain health: antioxidants and caffeine.

Caffeine offers several benefits to the brain, such as:

- **An increase in alertness:** caffeine blocks a chemical messenger called adenosine and helps keep you more alert. Adenosine is responsible for making you feel sleepy.

- **An improvement in your mood:** caffeine also boosts dopamine and other feel-good neurotransmitters.

- **Better concentration:** studies show that consuming caffeine enabled better alertness and attention over the short term in groups of people doing a cognition test.

Long-term consumption of coffee has also been linked to a reduction in the risk for neurological diseases, like Alzheimer's and Parkinson's, with the largest reduction in risk seen in people who consume three to four cups of coffee daily. This is partly down to the high antioxidant concentrations found in coffee.

3. Blueberries

It's long been known that blueberries are a superfood, offering plenty of health benefits for the body and some specifically targeting the brain. Like other deep-colored berries, blueberries contain anthocyanins, which are plant compounds packed with antioxidant and anti-inflammatory effects. Antioxidants fight inflammation and oxidative stress, both of which contribute to neurodegenerative diseases and brain aging.

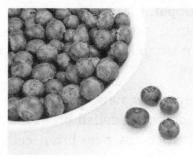

Wikimedia

Some of those antioxidants have been shown to build up in the brain over time, helping improve brain cell communication. One review of 11 separate studies concluded that blueberries help improve some cognitive processes and memory in adults and children.

Try adding blueberries to a smoothie or your bowl of oatmeal, or just snack on a few as they are.

4. Turmeric

Turmeric has suddenly found itself in the limelight as a health food, and this yellow-orange spice has long been used in curries. It also offers plenty of benefits for the brain. The active ingredient is curcumin, which has been shown to cross the blood-brain barrier, which means it has direct access to the brain and can provide benefits to the brain cells.

It has incredibly potent anti-inflammatory and antioxidant

properties, which have been linked to several benefits for the brain, including:

- **It can help memory:** curcumin can help improve the memory of those with Alzheimer's and can also help remove the amyloid plaques, a major indicator of the disease.

- **It can ease depression:** curcumin has been shown to boost two feel-good neurotransmitters that improve mood – dopamine and serotonin. A study showed that it helped improve the symptoms of anxiety and depression when it was used with standard prescribed treatments.

- **It can help grow new brain cells:** curcumin boosts a growth hormone called brain-derived neurotrophic factor, which helps new brain cells to grow. It may also help delay mental decline related to age, but more research needs to be done first.

However, you must remember that most research is done using highly concentrated doses of curcumin, in supplements ranging from 500 to 2000 mg per day. This is way more than you will consume by using turmeric in your kitchen because standard turmeric is only about 3 to 6% curcumin. So, although adding this spice to your food is beneficial, you might want to consider taking a curcumin supplement to get the real benefits – do consult your doctor first.

5. Broccoli

Broccoli is another superfood, packed with antioxidants and other plant compounds that benefit health. It has high levels of vitamin K, and a 160-gram (1 cup) serving provides more than the recommended daily allowance.

Vitamin K is fat-soluble and is crucial in forming sphingolipids, a densely packed fat in our brain cells. Studies in older people have shown that high vitamin K intake leads to better cognitive and memory status.

Broccoli also contains several antioxidant and anti-inflammatory compounds that can help protect the brain from being damaged.

6. Pumpkin Seeds

Pumpkin seeds are packed with antioxidants that help protect the brain and body from damage caused by free radicals. They also contain high levels of iron, magnesium, copper, and zinc, each of which plays its own part in brain health:

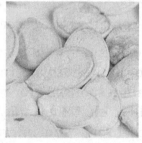

Wikimedia

- **Iron:** people who are deficient in iron often complain that their brain function is impaired, and they have brain fog.

- **Magnesium:** magnesium is critical for memory and learning, and low levels have been linked to depression, migraine, epilepsy, and other neurological diseases.

- **Copper:** copper is used to control the brain's nerve signals, and when you have a copper imbalance, you are at a high risk of Alzheimer's and other neurodegenerative diseases.

- **Zinc:** this is a crucial nerve signaling element, and

a zinc deficiency has been linked to Parkinson's, Alzheimer's, depression, and other neurological conditions.

Most of the research is done on these four micronutrients and not on the actual pumpkin seeds; however, because the seeds contain high levels of these four micronutrients, it follows that you can benefit from adding them to your diet.

7. Dark Chocolate

Cocoa powder and dark chocolate are high in several compounds that help boost the brain, including caffeine, flavonoids, and antioxidants. The best dark chocolate is that with a minimum of 70% cocoa content, and you don't get any of these benefits with milk chocolate, which contains little cocoa.

Flavonoids are plant compounds with antioxidant properties, and when you consume dark chocolate, those flavonoids gather in the parts of the brain responsible for memory and learning. Some researchers believe that they may help to slow down mental decline related to age and improve memory. Several studies have been shown to back this research.

One study on more than 900 people found that those who regularly ate dark chocolate performed better when asked to do mental tasks, including some that involved memory, than those who didn't eat much or any chocolate.

Research also shows that chocolate is legitimately an excellent mood booster, and a study showed that people who ate chocolate had more positive feelings than those who ate crackers. However, we can't be clear about whether that's because eating chocolate makes you feel happy or because of the flavonoids!

8. Nuts

Research shows that nuts are excellent for improving markers for heart health; a healthy heart is positively linked to a healthy brain. One study showed that when older adults consumed nuts regularly, they had a lower risk of cognitive decline.

Another study in 2014 determined that women who regularly consumed nuts over a few years had much sharper memories than those who never ate nuts.

Nuts contain several nutrients, including antioxidants, healthy fats, and vitamin E, and these may go some way toward explaining why they benefit brain health so much. Vitamin E protects against damage from free radicals, helping slow mental decline in later years.

All nuts are healthy, but walnuts are thought to be one of the best because they also contain anti-inflammatory properties in the form of omega-3 fatty acids.

9. Oranges

One medium orange provides almost 100% of the vitamin C you need in a day. This boosts brain health because vitamin C plays a key role in reducing the risks of mental decline. One study showed that higher levels of vitamin C in the blood led to an improvement in tasks where decision speed, attention, memory, and focus were required.

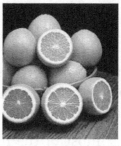

wikimedia

Vitamin C is one of the most powerful antioxidants in helping to fight free radicals and stop them from damaging your brain cells. Vitamin C also supports brain cells in older people and can help reduce the risks of schizophrenia, Alzheimer's, anxiety, and major depressive disorder.

Oranges aren't the only food with high levels of vitamin C; you can also get it from strawberries, tomatoes, guava, bell peppers, and kiwi.

10. Eggs

Eggs contain many brain health nutrients, including vitamins B6, vitamin b12, choline, and folate. Choline is used by your body to make acetylcholine, an important neurotransmitter in memory and mood regulation.

Some studies show that a higher choline intake is linked to good mental function and memory, but few people consume enough choline to make a difference. Eggs are the best way, given that the yolks contain highly concentrated amounts of choline.

Women should aim for 425 mg daily, and men should aim for 550 mg. 1 egg yolk contains 112 mg.

The B vitamins in eggs also play an important brain health role. First, they slow mental decline in older people because they lower homocysteine levels. This amino acid has tentative links to Alzheimer's and dementia. It has also been shown that a B12 and folate deficiency is linked to depression.

Older people with dementia often have a folate deficiency, and studies have shown that taking a folic acid supplement can significantly decrease the risk of age-related mental decline. Vitamin B12 also helps regulate the brain's sugar levels and synthesize brain chemicals.

Like the pumpkin seeds, most of the research is done on the

micronutrients, not the eggs themselves. However, when you consume eggs, you consume those nutrients, so eggs are an excellent addition to your diet.

11. Green Tea

Like coffee, green tea contains brain-boosting caffeine and has been shown to improve focus, memory, performance, and alertness. However, green tea also contains other components that help your brain.

L-theanine is an amino acid that can enter the brain by crossing the blood-brain barrier. Once there, it helps improve activity from a neurotransmitter called GABA, helping to relieve anxiety and promoting relaxation. L-theanine increases alpha-wave frequency in the brain, helping you relax but not be tired.

One study showed that because green tea contains L-theanine, it counteracts the stimulation provided by caffeine and helps you to relax.

Green tea also contains antioxidants and polyphenols that can help reduce the risks of Parkinson's and Alzheimer's and protect against mental decline. And some studies even show that green tea can improve your memory.

As you can see, several foods can contribute to brain health, and some, like the tea, coffee, fruits, and vegetables listed here, contain antioxidants that protect the brain from damage. Others, like eggs and nuts, are full of nutrients that support brain development and improve memory.

You can improve your brain health and overall health by adding these foods to your diet and you'll find some of them included in my recipes.

CHAPTER 7: HAVING
A CHEAT DAY

Sticking to healthy eating all the time is not always easy; everyone gets the odd craving or urge to eat something they shouldn't on occasion. Research has shown that the occasional cheat meal can be important and won't necessarily derail your efforts, depending on what you eat and how much.

So, why are cheat meals important, and how do they benefit your diet?

IT'S ALL ABOUT YOUR METABOLISM

We need to focus on two primary hormones – ghrelin and leptin.

Ghrelin tells you when you are hungry. A peptide hormone, ghrelin can increase in your body when you are on a low-calorie weight loss diet because low-calorie diets do not fill you up. The same applies to low-fat diets.

Leptin regulates appetite and controls how full you feel; it's how your brain knows to send the signal that you've eaten enough. Production of leptin is entirely dependent on your calorie intake. If you eat too many calories, your leptin production increases, while it decreases if you are in a calorie deficit.

- **Cheating can regulate these hormones**

We all know that to lose weight, we need to eat fewer calories than your body needs for normal functioning – this is known as TEE (total energy expenditure.)

However, the longer you are on a low-calorie diet, the more used to it your body gets, and it adapts, leading to a plateau where you no longer lose weight. If you consume one high-calorie, high-carbohydrate meal, it can kickstart your metabolism again and regulate the ghrelin and leptin hormones, encouraging your body to burn the calories and not adapt to a lower intake.

One study looked at three groups of healthy men who were not obese. Each group was put through four separate four-day periods, consuming the following:

1. Underfeeding – 70% of their TEE

2. Overfeeding – 130% of their TEE

3. Eucaloric diet – 100% of their TEE (baseline)

The study showed that leptin levels decreased when the men ate less than their TEE. However, when they ate more, their leptin returned to its normal production levels, proving that cheat meals help regulate these important hormones.

A similar study on women showed that when they increased carbohydrate intake, thus consuming more calories, leptin levels increased by up to 28%. It also shows that 24-hour energy expenditure improved by 7%, meaning that you burn more calories in a 24-hour period without needing to do any extra exercise.

CHEAT MEALS ARE MOTIVATING

What better way is there to keep you on your healthy diet than knowing you've got a wonderful cheat meal to look forward to?

How often you have a cheat meal depends on you. You should avoid cheating like the plague when starting your new diet or lifestyle. You need to give your body the best chance to get used to your new way of eating, but once you reach a plateau and get stuck on it for some time, you can consider cheating.

Some people say you should have a cheat meal a couple of times a week, but that seems excessive to me. If you tend to overeat, cheat meals are a definite no-no but if you must have one, make them few and far apart.

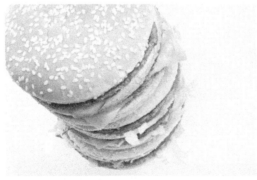

stockvault

Most people find that if they have a delicious meal to look forward to, they can stick to their diet and just know that meal will taste amazing, knowing that they've put in work to earn it.

Cheat meals also allow you a mental break, especially if you've been good for so long but are starting to struggle with cravings. It's exhausting, but by giving yourself a break once in a while, you can relax and enjoy your food.

If you follow my blog and try my recipes and lifestyle, you won't want to cheat, but if you feel like you want to, here are some tips on enjoying it without derailing your hard work.

HOW TO ENJOY A CHEAT MEAL

Now that you know how important cheat meals can be, we can look at ways to make it count but stay on track.

- **It's only a cheat meal, not the whole day**

This is a common mistake – people think they can cheat for an entire day. That is the easiest way to undo all your hard work, making it even harder to get back on track.

Cheat meals are not about grazing on an all-you-can-eat buffet; they are about compromise. If you have an all-or-nothing mindset, you cannot cheat on your diet – it won't work because you will eat more than you should. Think about the last time you has a slice or two of pizza. Did you have garlic bread, too, thinking it wouldn't make any difference? Well, it does, especially when you have to go back to your healthy eating regime.

Sure, enjoy a slice of pizza or even two, but don't go with all the extras. That way, you compromise – you stay sensible and accountable while satisfying a craving.

- **Only eat good quality food**

Another mistake people make on a cheat meal is to eat junk food. If you want a cheeseburger, have one but go for one made with a 100% beef burger, preferably grass-fed and free of hormones. If you want pizza, make it yourself – that way, you know what's going into your food. Do not make the mistake of binging on processed foods because they will undo everything you have achieved. Plus, keeping your cheat meal healthy will make it easier to get back to your healthy diet.

This even applies to dessert. If you want cookies, make them at home and use coconut flour, almond flour, or flaxseed meal rather than bleached white flour. If the recipe calls for sugar, swap it for coconut sugar or honey.

If you don't like cooking, you can still eat packaged foods, but check the labels and choose foods with the fewest amount of ingredients. That way, you know they are relatively healthy.

- **Keep it Balanced**

Studies show that high-carbohydrate cheat meals work best as they work better on leptin production than high-fat meals. However, you mustn't forget to balance those carbs with healthy fats and protein.

Many people feel guilty when eating a cheat meal and believe they will undo all their effort. You won't if you are sensible – you've worked for it, so enjoy it. Just be sensible, choose healthier options, and don't binge.

CHAPTER 8: THE BALANCE BETWEEN DIET AND EXERCISE

Diet is not the only factor in losing weight; exercise is also incredibly important for toning up your body, boosting your weight loss, and improving your health. Many people think they cannot or should not exercise while following an IF or low-carb lifestyle, but this is wrong.

When you first start following these lifestyles, it takes your body and mind time to get used to things. However, once you are in the swing of things, you should introduce some cardio and strength training to your plan – what you do is entirely down to what you enjoy doing. You should follow some tips to make things easier for you, though.

- **Ease into things**

Everyone is different, and no one plan suits all people. Build your workouts up slowly as your body adjusts to its new lifestyle. Working out for an hour is probably too much to start with, so begin with short sessions and build them up gradually.

- **Choose the right time**

If you are already used to working out in the morning, you'll need to change your eating window to ensure you eat a meal as soon as you finish your cardio. If you prefer to work out in the afternoons, that's a great time for weight training, while you can do low intensity training any time you want.

• Be flexible

While an eating window of noon to 8 PM might work for one person, it doesn't mean it will work for you. If you like going for a morning run, you'll need to consider changing your eating time to 9 AM to 5 PM to ensure you get a post-workout meal.

• Drink water

You may not be eating for several hours a day, but you still need to consume plenty of water. This is even more important if you intend to do fasted cardio, and you should try to consume a minimum of 72 ounces of water daily, a lot more if your workouts make you sweat heavily.

• Add electrolytes

Replenishing your electrolytes is important, whether you work out or not. To ensure you do this without breaking your fast, drink natural sports drinks or coconut water – do NOT opt for sugary drinks, sports or otherwise.

• Don't do the same workouts

Vary things; your body will respond better if you mix cardio and strength training. Not only will you be blasting the fat, but you'll also be building muscle. This works for your IF schedule – do your cardio when you can do morning workouts and focus on strength training when you need to exercise in the afternoon or evening. If you have no energy for strenuous exercise, skip it or do some gentle Pilates or yoga instead.

- **Let your body lead you**

Always listen to what your body is telling you because the best workout will be one that rejuvenates and strengthens you, not one that will leave you exhausted. Your body will tell you what it needs, so learn to listen to it and don't push yourself too hard just so you can do the exercise you think you should be doing rather than what you need to do.

What About Alternate-Day Fasting or 5:2?

If you choose a fasting plan that restricts your calories significantly on certain days, you should skip working out on those days or choose something low intensity. Never do anything that is likely to increase how many calories you expend on days when you need to conserve them because the more calories you burn, the further depleted your body becomes.

If you exercise on days when you are sticking to 500 calories, your body becomes depleted. That leaves you feeling exhausted and at a higher risk of injury, and you'll take longer to recover. Make sure your main workouts are on your higher calories days and rest up on the other days.

Play around and see what works best for you. And don't that IF isn't about not eating; it's about eating to a certain schedule, consuming the calories and nutrition you need only within a set window of time. You are not skipping meals; instead, you are eating them on a schedule, optimizing your food intake and getting the best results.

Most importantly, listen to what your body tells you.

HEALTHY FOODS FOR BASIC WORKOUTS

You need to feed your body with the right food to get the best of your performance when you exercise. This ensures you have enough stamina, can build up your strength, and your energy levels stay high. If you don't fuel up and prepare your body right, your recovery time will be much longer.

Try to include these power foods in your daily diet:

- **Banana**

These are perfect as a snack just before a workout, providing an excellent source of good carbohydrates that you need to maintain energy, and a high potassium level, which is needed for your muscles and nerves to function properly. You lose potassium when you sweat during your workout, so giving yourself extra before you start is beneficial.

- **Wholegrain Foods**

Exercise is an excellent way of raising your energy levels, but you also want plenty of that energy before you start. This is why you need certain carbohydrates, such as wholegrain foods. This includes wholegrain bread, brown rice, corn, and rolled oats, all low GI, which means they slowly release energy into your body.

- **Smoothies**

Smoothies are an excellent choice to drink just before a workout; there's a good reason for that. When making your smoothies, add a good mix of fruit (including berries and bananas), vegetables (especially green, leafy ones), whole yogurt, and even protein powder if you want. That gives you a great blend of minerals and vitamins, including vitamin C, calcium, and iron, all things that your body needs for great performance.

- **Lean Protein**

Protein is an essential building block, especially when you work out, as it helps your tissues and muscles repair. Good sources include salmon, turkey, chicken, tofu, nuts, and eggs.

- **Hummus**

Hummus is packed with carbohydrates, protein and unsaturated fats, great ingredients to help keep your energy levels high when you need it. Add a whole meal pitta or raw vegetables to get an all-round healthy snack.

FOOD FOR ADVANCED WORKOUTS

When your workouts are more intensive, you need to feed your body the right amount of protein to improve your fitness and maintain your health. Every cell in your body contains protein, and it has many roles, not least developing enzymes, producing hormones and other chemicals, and building and repairing body tissue. The human body requires a lot of protein because it can't make and draw on it when needed.

These four foods are packed with protein and make great snacks, both pre, and post-workout, and should be part of your daily diet:

- **Greek Yogurt**

Greek yogurt is one of the easiest foods to eat before your workout and is packed with calcium, probiotic bacteria to help your gut, and almost twice as much protein as regular yogurt. Add some fruit, granola, or other multigrain to give it a natural boost of sugar.

- **Poultry**

Chicken and turkey breast have high protein levels, perfect for helping you maintain your energy levels and build muscle during your workout. For a really healthy meal, add some steamed vegetables and brown rice.

- **Sardines**

People often overlook sardines, but they are full of omega-3 fatty acids and plenty of protein. They also contain a high level of vitamin D, which is needed to strengthen your bones. For a quick and easy snack, eat them on a slice of wholegrain toast, and choose the ones in tomato sauce if you can.

- **Nuts**

Nuts are a fantastic protein source and perfect for a quick snack before a workout. Have a small handful of cashews, peanuts, or other nuts for a burst of healthy unsaturated fat and protein, not to mention the zinc, potassium, calcium, and iron they contain. Buy unsalted nuts to avoid eating too much sodium.

FOODS TO AVOID

What you eat before a workout is crucial to how well your body performs, but by the same token, what you don't eat is also crucial. Some foods boost your energy, while others give you a short boost followed quickly by a slump – the last thing you want during a workout.

The five foods below should be avoided before a workout:

- **Spicy Foods**

Spicy food commonly leads to indigestion and heartburn, and you don't want either of these when you are working out. Not only will they make you uncomfortable, but they'll leave you feeling ill and result in your workout being cut short.

- **Refined Sugar**

We discussed refined sugar earlier, and many people think they should eat sugary foods before or after a workout to give them the energy they need. Sure, a candy bar might give you a boost, but it won't last long and will result in a slump that leaves you drained.

- **Artificial Sweeteners**

The same thing applies if you consume artificial sweeteners before your workout. These are mostly found in drinks, but some foods also have them, especially those labeled "sugar-free."

- **Fried Foods**

Fried food should be avoided anyway, as it's never good for you, but it's even worse for you if you eat it before a workout. Fried foods don't digest very easily and won't provide a slow, sustained energy release to get you through your workout. And it's a safe bet that if you work out after eating fried food, you won't feel too well.

- **Salt**

While working out, the last thing you want is to dehydrate because it can result in bad headaches. In extreme situations, it can also make you pass out. Avoid eating foods that are too salty, and drink plenty of water before, during, and after your workout session.

Too many people who work out tend to overlook their diet but giving your body the right type of fuel and the right amount will give you much better results, and the right food can make all the difference in your body's performance during the workout.

Now you know what you should and shouldn't eat, let's finish this book with some great, healthy recipes.

CHAPTER 9: DELICIOUS, EASY RECIPES

This is just a small selection of healthy, tasty and easy recipes that feed you and provide valuable nutrition throughout the day without feeling deprived of anything. You can find more recipes on my blog, Wander Culinaire and there are full step-by-step videos on my YouTube channel.

BREAKFAST

Easy Breakfast Salad

Ingredients:

- 1 medium-sized sweet potatoes, cut into cubes
- 0,5 large red bell pepper, cut into thin strips
- Extra virgin olive oil
- ½ teaspoon of chopped garlic
- ½ teaspoon of salt
- Ground black pepper to taste
- 2 cups of baby spinach, arugula, or another leafy green mix
- 1 egg
- 1 strips of cooked bacon, chopped coarsely

Directions:

1. Preheat your oven to 400°F
2. Lay baking paper over a large, lipped baking tray
3. Lay the bell pepper and sweet potato on the tray and drizzle with a tablespoon of olive oil. Season with salt, pepper, and garlic powder and toss to coat everything
4. Bake for about 20 to 25 minutes or until the potatoes are fork tender. Take them out of the oven and set them aside.
5. Cook the egg in a pan over medium heat, sunny-side-up
6. Mix the roasted vegetables between the greens, add a fried egg on top of each and sprinkle with bacon bits. You can also add slices of avocado for a boost of healthy fats.

Nutrition:

Serving: 1 salad

- **Calories:** 289
- **Sugar:** 5 g
- **Total Fat:** 19 g

- **Carbohydrates:** 18 g
- **Fiber:** 4 g
- **Protein:** 12 g
- **Cholesterol:** 186 mg

Mediterranean Avocado Toast

Ingredients:

- 1 egg
- 1 sliced tomato
- ½ a ripe avocado
- 0,5 clove garlic, finely chopped
- A handful of spinach or arugula
- A handful of fresh basil leaves
- ½ a green bell pepper, sliced into 4 or 5 strips
- 3 or 4 olives, sliced in half, pits removed
- 1 slice of whole-grain bread
- Ground black pepper

Directions:

1. Toast the bread to your preference and then leave it to cool
2. Prepare the egg to your preference – boiled, scrambled, fried, or poached.
3. Mash the avocado and mix in the garlic
4. Spread it over the toast evenly
5. Top off with slices of pepper and tomato, basil and spinach, and the olives
6. Season with black pepper, and then add the egg on top

Nutrition:

Serving: 1 slice of avocado toast

- **Calories:** 618
- **Sugar:** 29 g
- **Total Fat:** 25 g
- **Carbohydrates:** 87 g
- **Fiber:** 24 g
- **Protein:** 27 g
- **Cholesterol:** 186 mg

Healthy Overnight Oats

Ingredients:

- ½ cup old-fashioned oats
- 2 tablespoons of plain full-fat yogurt
- 1 teaspoon of chia seeds
- ¼ cup of water or milk of your choice
- 1 teaspoon of organic honey or maple syrup

For Vegan Oats:

- 1/3 cup of old-fashioned oats
- 1 tablespoon of chia seeds
- 1 teaspoon of organic honey or maple syrup
- ½ cup of cashew milk

Directions:

1. Place all the ingredients in a mixing bowl, mix them well together.
2. Leave them for a minute before stirring again, transfer in a Mason jar.
3. Seal the jar and refrigerate for at least 3 hours, preferably overnight
4. Add your choice of toppings before serving

Overnight oats go best with sweet toppings, such as:

- Fruit – sliced apples, bananas, berries, peaches, apricots, etc.
- Seeds and nuts
- Coconut shavings
- Nut butter (without sugar)

Nutrition:

Serving: 1 jar of oats

- **Calories:** 262
- **Sugar:** 22 g
- **Total Fat:** 7 g

- **Carbohydrates:** 46 g
- **Fiber:** 7 g
- **Protein:** 6 g
- **Cholesterol:** 0 mg

High Protein Lemon Blueberry Pancakes

Ingredients:

For the Pancakes:

- ½ cup of old-fashioned oats
- 3 egg whites
- 2 scoops of protein powder – vanilla flavor
- ½ cup of full-fat cottage cheese
- 2 teaspoons of lemon juice – freshly squeezed is best
- ¼ teaspoon of lemon zest
- ¼ cup of water
- 2/3 cup of fresh blueberries and extra for topping
- Coconut oil

For the Topping:

- ¼ cup of full-fat, plain Greek yogurt
- 1 tablespoon of organic honey
- 1 teaspoon of fresh lemon juice
- ¼ teaspoon of lemon zest

Directions:

1. Make the pancakes. Place the egg whites, oats, protein powder, cottage cheese, lemon juice, zest, and water in a blender
2. Blend to a puree – the protein powder will stick to the sides of the blender, so use a silicon spatula to scrape it into the mixture
3. Pour the puree into a bowl and fold the blueberries in gently
4. Heat a pan over medium-high heat, greasing it with a little coconut oil, about a teaspoon. More will be needed as you cook the pancakes
5. When the oil is hot, measure 1/3 of a cup of pancake mixture and pour it into the pan. Cook it for about 2 to 4 minutes, or until the edges are starting to get hard and a spatula slides easily beneath it

6. Flip the pancake and cook for a further 2 to 4 minutes or until the pancake batter is cooked through
7. Repeat until the batter is used up
8. Make the topping. Mix the honey, yogurt, juice, and zest in a bowl and drizzle over the pancakes.
9. Top off with a few fresh blueberries and a little extra lemon zest

Nutrition:

Serving: 1 pancake

- **Calories:** 185
- **Sugar:** 5.5 g
- **Total Fat:** 7.1 g
- **Carbohydrates:** 15.5 g
- **Fiber:** 2.3 g
- **Protein:** 14.8 g
- **Cholesterol:** 22.1 mg

Healthy Pancakes
Ingredients:

- 8 tbsp whole wheat flour
- 2 tsp baking powder
- 2 tsp coconut sugar
- 10 g protein powder
- 2 eggs
- A pinch of salt
- 100 ml of almond milk
- 10 g unsalted butter

For the Plating:

- 4 whole strawberries
- 200 g of Papaya
- 1 tbsp full-fat plain Greek yogurt
- 1 tbsp organic maple syrup
- 2 whole mint leaves

Instructions:

1. Make the pancake dough. Put the flour, baking powder, sugar, eggs, protein powder, salt, and almond milk in the blender.
2. Blend until it's a smooth consistency
3. Melt the butter in the frying pan
4. Scoop a spoonful of pancake dough into the pan and cook for a few minutes until golden brown; flip and cook the other side.
5. Repeat for all the batter – you should get about 6 small pancakes

To Plate:

1. Peel the papaya and slice it into wedges.
2. Rinse the strawberries, remove the leaves, and slice

them in half

3. Arrange the pancakes on a plate with the papaya slices. Add the strawberries and mint to the side and top the pancakes with Greek yogurt and a swirl of maple syrup.

Nutrition per Serving (1 serving):

- **Calories:** 251 kcal
- **Carbohydrate:** 44 g
- **Protein:** 10 g
- **Fat:** 6 g
- **Saturated Fat:** 3 g
- **Polyunsaturated Fat:** 1 g
- **Monounsaturated Fat:** 2 g
- **Trans Fats:** 0.2 g
- **Cholesterol:** 23 mg
- **Sodium:** 573 mg
- **Potassium:** 344 mg
- **Fiber:** 5 g
- **Sugar:** 17 g
- **Vitamin A:** 1139 UI
- **Vitamin C:** 62 mg
- **Calcium:** 368 mg
- **Iron:** 2 mg

Shakshouka
Ingredients:

- 4 pearl onions
- 2 cloves of garlic
- 4 whole mushrooms
- 3 fresh tomatoes or unsweetened canned tomatoes
- ½ a red bell pepper
- 1 tsp extra virgin olive oil
- A pinch of salt
- 1 tsp dried cilantro
- 1 tsp paprika powder
- ½ a chili
- 100 ml of water
- 2 eggs

For the Garnish:

- 1 whole grain unsweetened pita bread
- 1 tsp cilantro
- 1 tsp tahini

Instructions:

1. Finely chop the tomato, mushrooms, bell pepper, garlic, and onions. Remove the seeds from the chili pepper

2. Heat a pan and add the olive oil. Sauté the onion, mushrooms, bell pepper, and garlic, seasoned with salt. When the vegetables have softened, add the tomatoes and a small amount of water

3. Add the chili, stir, and cook for about 15 minutes, stirring occasionally

4. Break the eggs into the mixture and poach them as you like them; for example, medium hard poached eggs will take about 5 to 10 minutes.

5. To serve, warm the pita bread in the oven. Dish the shakshuka onto plates, swirl the tahini over the top and add cilantro leaves to garnish.

Nutrition per Serving (1 serving):

- **Calories:** 89 kcal
- **Carbohydrate:** 5 g
- **Protein:** 2 g
- **Fat:** 7 g
- **Saturated Fat:** 1 g
- **Polyunsaturated Fat:** 2 g
- **Monounsaturated Fat:** 4 g
- **Cholesterol:** 7 mg
- **Sodium:** 56 mg
- **Potassium:** 129 mg
- **Fiber:** 1 g
- **Sugar:** 1 g
- **Vitamin A:** 1043 IU
- **Vitamin C:** 5 mg
- **Calcium:** 30 mg
- **Iron:** 1 mg

SMOOTHIES, SOUPS, AND SALADS

Spinach and Watermelon Salad

Ingredients:

For the Salad:

- 4 cups of fresh arugula or baby spinach
- 3 cups of watermelon, seedless or deseeded, cubed
- 2 cups of cantaloupe melon, cubed
- 2 cups of English cucumber, cubed
- ½ cup of fresh mint, roughly chopped
- 2 chopped green onions

For the Dressing:

- ¼ cup of white wine vinegar or rice vinegar
- 2 tablespoons of freshly squeezed lime juice
- 1 tablespoon of lime zest
- 2 tablespoons of olive oil
- 2 chopped garlic cloves
- 4 teaspoons of fresh ginger root, chopped
- ½ teaspoon of salt
- ¼ teaspoon of organic honey
- ¼ teaspoon of ground black pepper

Directions:

1. Combine the salad ingredients in a large bowl
2. Combine the dressing ingredients in another bowl, whisking to combine
3. Drizzle the dressing over the salad and serve

Nutrition:

Serving: 1 salad

- **Calories:** 84
- **Total Fat:** 4 g
- **Carbohydrates:** 13 g
- **Fiber:** 1 g
- **Protein:** 1 g

- **Cholesterol:** 288 mg

Bean and Shrimp Stew

Ingredients:

Shrimp Broth:

- 8 whole shrimp
- 1 tsp olive oil
- 1 tomato
- ½ carrot
- 2 pearl onions
- 1 whole garlic clove
- 2 tbsp low-sodium soy sauce
- 1 tbsp celery
- 2 g salt
- 600 ml water

Bean Stew:

- ½ a carrot, diced
- ½ an onion, diced
- 1 can of sugar-free white beans
- 2 tbsp chopped celery
- 1 tsp olive oil
- 1 tbsp basil
- 8 extra jumbo shrimp, cleaned
- 2 g salt

Instructions:

1. First, make the broth. Clean the shrimp (see my video on YouTube), retaining the shells and heads.
2. Heat a pot and toast the shells and heads. Add the water, tomato, salt, soy sauce, and onions, and stir.
3. Leave it to simmer slowly for about 45 minutes, occasionally spooning the foam off the top. When cooked, strain the broth into a separate bowl,

discarding the solids.

4. Next, make the bean stew. Sauté the onion and carrot and add the broth. Bring it to a boil and simmer on low for about 10 minutes or until the carrots are cooked.

5. Rinse and drain the beans and add them to the broth.

6. Add the basil and celery, and stir it in.

7. Heat the olive oil in a frying pan and cook the prawns. Season with salt and add a little butter if you like.

8. Transfer the bean stew to bowls, add the shrimp on top, and garnish with fresh basil.

Nutrition per Serving (1 serving):

- **Calories:** 302 kcal
- **Carbohydrate:** 48 g
- **Protein:** 19 g
- **Fat:** 5 g
- **Saturated Fat:** 1 g
- **Polyunsaturated Fat:** 1 g
- **Monounsaturated Fat:** 3 g
- **Cholesterol:** 6 mg
- **Sodium:** 8792 mg
- **Potassium:** 1067 mg
- **Fiber:** 11 g
- **Sugar:** 1 g
- **Vitamin A:** 158 UI
- **Vitamin C:** 1 mg
- **Calcium:** 185 mg
- **Iron:** 7 mg

Green Power Smoothie

Ingredients:

- ½ a frozen peach
- ½ a frozen banana
- 1 teaspoon of grated fresh ginger root
- ½ a large cucumber or 1 small one
- 1 cup of baby spinach
- 1/3 cup of almond milk
- Soaked chia seeds – optional

Directions:

1. Chop the peach, banana, and cucumber. You can use fresh but frozen fruit provides a much nicer, creamier consistency.
2. Add all the ingredients to the blender, except the chia, and blend to a smooth consistency
3. Add the soaked chia seeds if you are using them
4. Pour into a glass and enjoy

Nutrition:

Serving: 1 smoothie

- **Calories:** 153
- **Sugar:** 18 g
- **Total Fat:** 1 g
- **Carbohydrates:** 35 g
- **Fiber:** 8 g
- **Protein:** 8 g
- **Cholesterol:** 0 mg

Blueberry Smoothie Bowl

Ingredients:

- 1 cup of frozen blueberries
- ½ cup of almond milk, unsweetened
- 1 ½ scoops of vanilla protein powder
- 2 tablespoons of almond butter, unsweetened
- 1 teaspoon of pure vanilla extract or fresh one (more expensive)
- ½ cup of fresh blueberries
- ¼ cup of vanilla granola (sugar free), better make your own
- 2 tablespoons of sliced raw almonds
- 2 teaspoons of hemp seeds
- 1 teaspoon of ground cinnamon

Directions:

1. Place the frozen blueberries, protein powder, almond milk, vanilla extract, and almond butter in a blender and blend to a creamy consistency.
2. Divide the mixture equally between two small bowls.
3. Top off with granola, fresh blueberries, hemp seeds, sliced almonds, and cinnamon to serve.

Nutrition:

Serving: 2 bowls

- **Calories:** 370
- **Sugar:** 16 g
- **Total Fat:** 17 g
- **Carbohydrates:** 32 g
- **Fiber:** 7 g
- **Protein:** 25 g
- **Cholesterol:** 0 mg

Cheesy Chicken And Vegetable Salad

Ingredients:

- 1 cup of skinless and boneless chicken breast, cooked, chopped into cubes
- ¼ cup of finely chopped celery
- ¼ cup of raw carrot, shaved into strips
- ½ cup of roughly chopped baby spinach
- 4 tablespoons of yogurt
- 1/8 teaspoon of parsley
- 2 teaspoons of Dijon mustard
- ¼ cup of shredded cheddar cheese

Directions:

1. Place all the ingredients in a bowl and stir, coating everything in yogurt
2. Chill for 30 minutes or more before serving

Nutrition:

Serving: 1 salad

- **Calories:** 364.5
- **Sugar:** 7.3 g
- **Total Fat:** 9.1 g
- **Carbohydrates:** 15.3 g
- **Fiber:** 2.8 g
- **Protein:** 53.2 g
- **Cholesterol:** 131.8 mg

Avocado Chicken Salad

Ingredients:

- 4 ounces of cooked chicken breast
- ½ a large avocado
- 1 Hard-boiled egg
- 1/3 cup of chopped tomato
- ½ cup chopped spinach
- 1 to 2 thinly sliced scallions
- 1 chopped cucumber
- 1 tablespoon of chopped pitted olives
- Salt and pepper to season

For the Dressing:

- 1 tablespoon of extra virgin olive oil
- 1 clove of chopped garlic
- 1 tablespoon of freshly squeezed lemon juice
- 1 teaspoon of sesame oil – optional

Directions:

1. Make the salad. Place the spinach in a bowl and layer with tomatoes, cucumber, and avocado. Add the olives and chicken, slices of boiled egg, and sprinkle with the scallion. Season with pepper.
2. Make the dressing. Combine all the ingredients, whisking to a smooth consistency, and season with salt.
3. Drizzle the dressing over the salad and serve.

Nutrition:

Serving: 1 salad

- **Calories:** 635
- **Sugar:** 6 g
- **Total Fat:** 43 g
- **Carbohydrates:** 22 g
- **Fiber:** 12 g

- **Protein:** 44 g
- **Cholesterol:** 272 mg

Chickpea, Tomato, and Garlic Salad

Ingredients:

- ½ cup of canned chickpeas, no sugar added
- 1 small to medium green bell pepper
- 5 chopped olives
- 1 cup of arugula
- 3 medium tomatoes
- 3 to 4 mint leaves – optional
- 1 clove of garlic
- Extra virgin olive oil
- Salt and pepper
- Fresh lemon juice

Directions:

1. Drain the chickpeas and rinse them
2. Chop the pepper, olives, tomato, mint, and arugula, and chop the garlic
3. You can add the garlic directly to the other ingredients or add it to some olive and let it infuse for half an hour. If you choose that option, remove the garlic from the oil and just use the flavored oil
4. Place the chickpeas and vegetables in a large bowl and squeeze some fresh lemon juice; season to taste and serve.

Nutrition:

Serving: 1 salad

- **Calories:** 385
- **Sugar:** 17 g
- **Total Fat:** 19 g
- **Carbohydrates:** 48 g
- **Fiber:** 15 g
- **Protein:** 13 g
- **Cholesterol:** 0 mg

Mediterranean Salmon Salad

Ingredients:

- 4 ounces of steamed salmon fillet
- 2 cups of cabbage
- 1 cup of arugula
- ½ cup of cherry tomatoes
- ½ cup of cucumber
- 1 scallion
- 1 chopped garlic clove
- 1 tablespoon of extra virgin olive oil
- 1 teaspoon of fresh lemon juice
- 2 tablespoons of feta cheese
- 2 small radishes
- 1 red pepper, roasted
- Salt and pepper to season

Directions:

1. If your salmon is uncooked, steam it for 10 minutes to cook it first.
2. Chop the tomatoes, radishes, scallion, cucumber, and cabbage and place them in a large bowl
3. Flake the salmon and crumble the cheese. Add them to the bowl and season to taste.

Nutrition:

Serving: 1 salad

- **Calories:** 584
- **Sugar:** 18 g
- **Total Fat:** 36 g
- **Carbohydrates:** 33 g
- **Fiber:** 9 g
- **Protein:** 36 g
- **Cholesterol:** 92 mg

Coconut Curry Shrimp Soup

Ingredients:

- 400 ml of unsweetened coconut milk
- ½ chopped zucchini
- 6 ounces of deveined and peeled shrimp
- 5 lime leaves or some lemon grass
- 1 ½ teaspoons of red curry paste
- A handful of chopped fresh cilantro

Direction:

1. Roast the curry paste slightly in a large pan and add the coconut milk. Stir to combine and cook over medium-high heat. Keep stirring until the mixture is smooth and even. Add the lemongrass or lime leaves.
2. Add the shrimp and cook until the shrimp has turned pink
3. Stir the zucchini in and turn off the heat.
4. Fish out the lime leaves and serve garnished with fresh cilantro.
5. You can serve the curry with a cooked brown rice on the side.

Nutrition:

Serving:

- **Calories:** 358
- **Sugar:** 1 g
- **Total Fat:** 29 g
- **Carbohydrates:** 13 g
- **Fiber:** 1 g
- **Protein:** 17 g
- **Cholesterol:** 120 mg

Berry, Chia, and Mint Smoothie

Ingredients:

- 1 cup of sliced fresh strawberries
- ½ cup of fresh raspberries
- ½ cup of beetroot, without skin
- 1/3 cup of mint leaves
- 1 tablespoon of chia seeds
- 1 cup of unsweetened almond milk

Directions:

1. Add the beetroot, mint, berries, and chia seeds into a freezer-safe jar or Ziploc bag and freeze overnight, preferably longer.
2. When you are ready to prepare the smoothie, add the milk to a blender. Place the frozen ingredients in the blender and blend to a smooth consistency.
3. Serve in two glasses.

Nutrition:

Serving: 2 glasses

- **Calories:** 105
- **Sugar:** 7 g
- **Total Fat:** 3.5 g
- **Carbohydrates:** 17 g
- **Fiber:** 8 g
- **Protein:** 3 g
- **Cholesterol:** 0 mg

MAIN MEALS

Pumpkin with Feta Cheese and Walnuts

Ingredients:

- 5 lbs. pumpkin, deseeded, peeled, and chopped into cubes about 1-inch square
- ¼ cup extra virgin olive oil, divided
- 2 teaspoons of salt
- 1 teaspoon of pepper
- 2 medium onions, chopped
- 2/3 cup of roughly chopped walnuts
- 2/3 cup of feta cheese, crumbled
- 20 thin sliced fresh sage leaves

Directions:

1. Preheat your oven to 375°F
2. Grease a baking tray, 15 x 1 x 1 inch, and place the pumpkin in it. Drizzle 2 tablespoons of the oil over the pumpkin and season it with salt and pepper. Bake it until tender, about 30 to 35 minutes.
3. Meanwhile, heat the remaining oil in a large skillet and sauté the onions until they are tender. Add the walnuts and toast them for about 3 to 5 minutes.
4. Remove the pumpkin from the onion, place it on a serving platter, and top it off with the onion and walnuts. Scatter feta cheese and sage over the top and serve.

Nutrition:

Serving: 1 bowl

- **Calories:** 154
- **Sugar:** 4 g
- **Total Fat:** 11 g
- **Carbohydrates:** 12 g
- **Fiber:** 2 g
- **Protein:** 4 g
- **Cholesterol:** 6 mg

Cabbage and Ground Beef Stir-Fry

Ingredients:

- 3 cups of cabbage – red or green, your choice
- 2 finely chopped scallions
- 1 finely chopped red pepper
- 2 minced garlic cloves
- 1 ½ tablespoons of tamari sauce (a thicker Japanese version of a soy sauce)
- 1 tablespoon of olive oil
- 3 tablespoons of chopped cilantro or parsley
- 8 ounces of ground beef
- 1 carrot, sliced into thin strips
- 2 teaspoons of crushed red pepper

Directions:

1. Add the beef, a clove of minced garlic, and a little oil of your choice to a pan and heat over medium-high heat. Stir it after a minute, breaking the beef up, and then let it sauté for about 5 or 6 minutes.
2. Meanwhile, chop up the vegetables and stir the cabbage, carrots, scallions, and one more clove of garlic into the beef. Cover the pan and cook it for about 2 or 3 minutes, or until the vegetables are cooked,
3. Stir the peppers and remaining garlic clove in, add the tamari sauce, and stir, cooking for another 2 or 3 minutes – add a little more oil if you need to.
4. Turn the heat off and stir the parsley in before serving.

Nutrition:

Serving: 1 plate

- **Calories:** 472
- **Sugar:** 10 g
- **Total Fat:** 27 g
- **Carbohydrates:** 23 g
- **Fiber:** 7 g

- **Protein:** 37 g
- **Cholesterol:** 101 mg

Tandoori Meatballs with Spicy Carrot Mash

Ingredients:

- 2/3 cup of thick Greek yogurt, plus a bit extra for serving
- 2 ½ tablespoons of tandoori paste
- 23 ounces of lean, ground minced beef
- 1 tablespoon of tomato paste
- 2 tablespoons of chopped fresh coriander
- A 3 cm piece of fresh ginger root, grated
- 3 crushed garlic cloves
- 3 thickly sliced carrots
- 1 tablespoon of extra virgin olive oil
- Juice from a lemon
- 1 teaspoon of ground cinnamon
- 1 teaspoon of ground cumin
- 1 ½ cups of frozen peas
- ¼ bunch of fresh mint, leaves picked off

Directions:

1. Preheat your oven to 350°F and place a sheet of baking paper on a baking tray
2. Mix the yogurt, tandoori paste, and tomato paste in a bowl and season it
3. Use your hands to combine the minced beef, ginger, coriander, and garlic in a bowl. Roll the mixture into 16 balls and coat them in the yogurt sauce.
4. Place the meatballs on the baking tray and cook for about 20 to 25 minutes or until cooked through.
5. In the meantime, cook the carrot in a pot of salted boiling water for about 10 minutes or until tender. Drain the carrots and put them back in the pan with the spices, lemon juice, and oil. Mash the carrots and season.
6. Cook the peas in salted boiling water for a minute and drain.

7. Serve the meatballs with carrot mash, peas, and mint leaves, with extra yogurt on the side.

Nutrition:

Serving: 1 bowl

- **Calories:** 404
- **Total Fat:** 19.3 g
- **Carbohydrates:** 13.3 g
- **Fiber:** 7 g
- **Protein:** 40.5 g
- **Cholesterol:** 109 mg

SNACKS AND DESSERTS

Healthy Apple Crumble

Ingredients:

- 2 sweet apples
- 1 teaspoon of coconut oil
- 1 teaspoon of ground cinnamon
- ½ cup of old-fashioned oats
- ¼ cup of raw nuts
- 1 teaspoon of organic honey
- 1 tablespoon of shredded coconut unsweetened
- 1 ½ tablespoons of coconut oil
- 1 teaspoon of water
- 1 teaspoon of cinnamon
- A pinch of salt

Directions:

1. Core the apples, peel them, and cut them into cubes. Heat some coconut oil in a pan over medium heat and add some cinnamon. Stir in the apples and sauté them for a few minutes until they are coated in the oil and cinnamon. Cover the pan, and leave the apples to soften for a few minutes, adding a little water if needed.
2. Place the oats, nuts, honey, cinnamon, and shredded coconut in a food processor with the coconut oil. Pulse the mixture until you get a crumbly mixture; when you press it together with your fingers, it should stick.
3. Add half a tablespoon of coconut oil to a pan over medium-high heat and flatten the crumble mixture with a spatula. Heat the mixture for about 5 minutes, occasionally stirring, until it is golden brown. Remove it from the heat and let the crumble cool to a crispy consistency.
4. Place the apples in a bowl, top off with crumble, and serve as is or with yogurt, milk, or nut butter.

Nutrition:

Serving: 1 bowl

- **Calories:** 276
- **Sugar:** 16 g
- **Total Fat:** 16 g
- **Carbohydrates:** 33 g
- **Fiber:** 6 g
- **Protein:** 4 g
- **Cholesterol:** 0 mg

Easy Chia Pudding

Ingredients:

- 2 tablespoons of chia seeds
- ½ a teaspoon of organic honey or maple syrup
- ½ a cup of cashew or unsweetened almond milk
- Vanilla

For the Topping:

- Fresh berries of your choice
- 1 teaspoon of almond butter
- Chopped nuts – optional

Directions:

1. Put the chia seeds, honey/maple syrup, and vanilla in a mixing bowl and add the milk. Stir it until the chia seeds no longer clump.
2. Place the lid on the jar and refrigerate overnight.
3. Serve topped with berries, almond butter, and nuts.

Nutrition:

Serving: 1 jar

- **Calories:** 254
- **Sugar:** 16 g
- **Total Fat:** 10 g
- **Carbohydrates:** 33 g
- **Fiber:** 8 g
- **Protein:** 8 g
- **Cholesterol:** 10 mg

Mini Bacon and Spinach Quiches

Ingredients:

- 6 eggs
- 3 tablespoons of milk of your choice
- ¾ cup of spinach, chopped finely
- 1 cup of shredded cheddar cheese
- 4 strips of cooked bacon, chopped
- A pinch of pepper

Directions:

1. Preheat your oven to 350°F and grease up a 24-count mini muffin tin.
2. Whisk the milk and eggs in a bowl and add the spinach, cheese, bacon, and pepper, stirring to combine.
3. Divide the mixture equally between the muffin cups and bake for about 15 to 18 minutes.
4. Remove the quiches from the oven and leave them to cool before removing them from the muffin cups.

Nutrition:

Serving: 1 mini quiche

- **Calories:** 47
- **Total Fat:** 3.5 g
- **Carbohydrates:** 0 g
- **Fiber:** 0 g
- **Protein:** 3.5 g
- **Cholesterol:** 53 mg

Vegan Shortbread Cookies

Ingredients:

- 1 cup of almond flour
- 1 cup of quick oats
- 2 ½ tablespoons of organic maple syrup
- 2 ½ tablespoons of coconut oil
- A pinch of salt

For the Almond Butter Topping:

- 2 tablespoons of almond butter
- ½ teaspoon of organic maple syrup
- A pinch of salt

For the Chocolate Topping:

- 2 tablespoons of dark chocolate
- 1 teaspoon of almond butter

Directions:

1. Preheat the oven to 350°F
2. Blend the cookie ingredients using a hand or regular blender.
3. Use clean, damp hands to shape the cookie dough into cookies and place each one on o greased, lined baking tray
4. Bake until golden brown, about 12 to 15 minutes.
5. Meanwhile, make the toppings. For the chocolate topping, melt the chocolate in the microwave for 30 seconds and stir in the almond butter.
6. Mix the butter with the syrup and salt to make the almond butter topping.
7. Remove the cookies from the oven and leave them to cool.
8. Top each one with almond butter topping, followed by chocolate topping
9. Refrigerate for 30 minutes to an hour before serving.

Nutrition:

Serving: 1 cookie

- **Calories:** 140
- **Sugar:** 4 g
- **Total Fat:** 10 g
- **Carbohydrates:** 10 g
- **Fiber:** 2 g
- **Protein:** 3 g
- **Cholesterol:** 0 mg

Banana Protein Muffins

Ingredients:

- 2 large bananas, over-ripe
- 1 large egg
- ¼ cup of organic honey or maple syrup
- ¼ cup smooth peanut butter
- 1 teaspoon of pure vanilla extract
- 1 teaspoon of cinnamon
- 1 teaspoon of baking powder
- 2 teaspoons of baking soda
- ¾ cup of almond flour
- ¼ cup of oat flour
- ¾ cup of plain whey protein powder
- 1 cup of fresh strawberries plus a few extra for garnish
- ¼ cup of mini chocolate chips plus 1 tablespoon for garnish
- Cooking spray

Directions:

1. Preheat your oven to 350°F and line a 12-count muffin pan with muffin cup liners, sprayed with some cooking spray.
2. Mash the banana in a large bowl and add the egg, peanut butter, maple syrup protein powder, extract,

baking powder, cinnamon, and baking soda. Whisk to a smooth, combined consistency.

3. Add the oat and almond flour, stirring them until well combined.
4. Chop a cup of strawberries into small pieces and stir them into the mixture with a cup of chocolate chips.
5. Divide the batter equally between the muffin cups and place more chopped strawberries and chocolate chips on top.
6. Bake for about 22 minutes – insert a toothpick into the center of one; it should come out clean. If not, cook them for a little longer but do not overbake them.
7. Remove the muffins from the oven and leave them to cool for about 15 minutes.

Nutrition:

Serving: 1 muffin

- **Calories:** 178
- **Sugar:** 11 g
- **Total Fat:** 8 g
- **Carbohydrates:** 18 g
- **Fiber:** 2 g
- **Protein:** 10 g
- **Cholesterol:** 25 mg

CONCLUSION

Thank you for taking the time to read my short guide. Many people think dieting is the answer to their problems, but, in reality, it's the diets causing the problems. Most diets only work in the short term; over the long term, they can lead to serious psychological and physical problems.

Too many people get caught up in the vicious cycle of yo-yo dieting. When one diet doesn't give them the desired results quickly, they try another, and another, and so on, until they suddenly realize that they weigh more than they did before they started – how did that happen?

Dieting isn't the answer. Acceptance of our natural bodies is the starting point; when we can do that, we can rebuild our relationship with food. We can learn how to eat properly without depriving ourselves and feed our bodies the nutrition they so desperately need to function properly.

If we can't do this, we will continue to cause significant harm to our health, making us unhappy; unhappiness leads to poor eating choices, making us even more unhappy – it's a tough cycle to get out of.

Hopefully, this guide, my blog, and YouTube channel will help you regain your confidence and rebuild your relationship with food, resulting in you being in a happy place and tip-top health.

Last, but not least, if this book values you and I could help you to get some insides of my food habits, it would be great if you share your experience with others. As my goal is to reach out and help as many people as possible!

Feel free to share your feedback with a review on Amazon.

Much success for your journey and NEVER GIVE UP!

Matthias

References

"6 Amazing Body Changes When You Give up Carbs." *Time*, time.com/4021985/simple-carbohydrates/.

"11 Best Foods to Boost Your Brain and Memory." *Healthline*, 9 May 2017, www.healthline.com/nutrition/11-brain-foods#TOC_TITLE_HDR_13.

"13 Simple Ways to Stop Eating Lots of Sugar." *Healthline*, 6 June 2021, www.healthline.com/nutrition/14-ways-to-eat-less-sugar#TOC_TITLE_HDR_16. Accessed 9 Nov. 2022.

"15 Benefits of Drinking Water and Other Water Facts." *Www.medicalnewstoday.com*, 16 July 2018, www.medicalnewstoday.com/articles/290814#kidney_damage.

Czarnecka, Kamila, et al. "Aspartame—True or False? Narrative Review of Safety Analysis of General Use in Products." *Nutrients*, vol. 13, no. 6, 1 June 2021, p. 1957, www.mdpi.com/2072-6643/13/6/1957, 10.3390/nu13061957.

Gunnars, Kris. "Intermittent Fasting 101 — the Ultimate Beginner's Guide." *Healthline*, Healthline Media, 25 July 2018, www.healthline.com/nutrition/intermittent-fasting-guide#should-you.

"HOME." *Wander Culinaire*, wanderculinaire.com/. Accessed 8 Nov. 2022.

Montgomery, Lorena. "Top Zucker Konsumierende Nationen Der Welt | 2022." *Ripleybelieves.com*, www.ripleybelieves.com/top-sugar-consuming-nations-in-world-3498. Accessed 10 Nov. 2022.

read, Dr Sarah Jarvis MBE20-Sep-17 · 6 mins. "How to Balance Your Exercise and Diet." *Patient.info*, patient.info/news-and-features/balancing-exercise-and-your-diet. Accessed 9 Nov. 2022.

Sisson, Mark. "Benefits of Pairing Low-Carb Eating with Intermittent Fasting for Health and Weight Loss." *Mark's Daily Apple*, 22 Jan. 2020, www.marksdailyapple.com/benefits-of-pairing-low-carb-eating-with-intermittent-fasting-for-health-and-weight-loss/. Accessed 9 Nov. 2022.

Trinh, Emily. "How Cheat Meals Can Actually Benefit Your Diet." *Aaptiv*, Aaptiv, 17 Dec. 2017, aaptiv.com/magazine/benefits-of-cheat-meals.

"Why Diets Don't Work." *Www.nutritionist-Resource.org.uk*, www.nutritionist-resource.org.uk/blog/2020/10/02/why-diets-dont-work#accept-cookies. Accessed 8 Nov. 2022.

Made in the USA
Monee, IL
21 August 2024

64308824R00095